CHIA

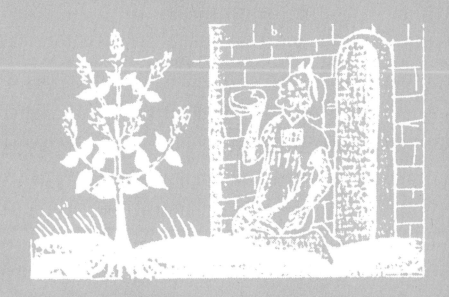

CHIA

Rediscovering a Forgotten Crop of the Aztecs

Ricardo Ayerza Jr. and Wayne Coates

THE UNIVERSITY OF ARIZONA PRESS

TUCSON

The University of Arizona Press
© 2005 The Arizona Board of Regents
All rights reserved

www.uapress.arizona.edu

Library of Congress Cataloging-in-Publication Data
appear on the last printed page of this book.

Manufactured in the United States of America on acid-free, archival-quality paper containing a minimum of 30% post-consumer waste and processed chlorine free.

13 12 11 10 09   7 6 5 4 3

Uei Tocoztli

In the *cu* of the courtyard they made from dough which they call *tzoalli*

the image of this goddess, and in front of her they offered all kinds

of maize, beans, and chia, because they said that she was the

source and bearer of those goods which are sustenance for

the people's life.

FRAY BERNARDINO DE SAHAGÚN,

HISTORIA GENERAL DE LAS COSAS

DE NUEVA ESPAÑA

CONTENTS

ILLUSTRATIONS

Figures

Tables

FOREWORD

Ing. Ricardo Ayerza Jr. and Dr. Wayne Coates, two outstanding scientists, provide in this work the most up-to-date information on the anthropological, historical, political, agricultural, and nutritional aspects of chia. Since chia seeds contain more alpha-linolenic acid (63 percent) than any other seed, the authors present an extensive discussion of the role of omega-3 fatty acids and the importance of the omega-6 to omega-3 fatty acid ratio in health and disease.

Human beings evolved on a diet that was balanced in the omega-6 to omega-3 fatty acid ratio. Prior to the development of agribusiness the two families of omega-6 and omega-3 essential fatty acids were found throughout the food supply: in meat, milk and other dairy products, fish, legumes, plants, and fruit. Modern agribusiness led to changes in animal feeds. In the past animals and poultry grazed and thus obtained both omega-6 and omega-3 fatty acids from grasses. But today animals are grain-fed, mostly corn, which is high in omega-6 fatty acids. Thus beef and dairy products from grain-fed cattle do not contain any omega-3 fatty acids. In a study conducted in Greece my colleagues and I showed that under natural conditions eggs from chickens that graze have a ratio of omega-6 to omega-3 of 1:3, whereas the standard United States Department of Agriculture egg has a ratio of omega-6 to omega-3 of about 20:1 (Simopoulos and Salem, 1992).

Our egg, known as the Greek egg or Ampelistra egg, from a farm in Greece where the chickens fetch their own food by grazing, is now considered the "standard natural" egg for omega-3 enrichment. Changing chicken feed by adding omega-3 fatty acids from fish meal or flaxseed (both good sources of omega-3 fatty acids) has made omega-3 enriched eggs available throughout the world. Because omega-3 fatty acids are essential for normal growth and development and in the treatment of coronary heart disease, mental health problems, arthritis, and other chronic diseases, it is now recognized that there is a need to return omega-3 fatty acids into the food supply.

Chia was one of the main foods of both the Aztec and the Mayan diet and presents an opportunity to improve human nutrition by providing a natural, plant-based source of omega-3 fatty acids, antioxidants, and dietary fiber. Chia seed, with the highest content of alpha-linolenic acid of known plants, is an excellent source to enrich eggs with omega-3 fatty acids as well as poultry meat, pork, milk, and so on. Ayerza and Coates's research has contributed immensely in this regard. Their book is a major contribution to nutrition research and to the return of omega-3 fatty acids into the food supply.

Artemis P. Simopoulos, M.D.
Center for Genetics, Nutrition and Health
Washington, D.C.

CHIA

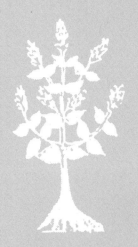

ONE

The Paradox of Hunger and Abundance

The Green Revolution

In 1970 Dr. Norman Borlaug received the Nobel Peace Prize for his contributions to solving the problem of world hunger. His work was aimed at meeting the basic needs of the people of the world by increasing production of traditional crops such as wheat and corn. His success is clear and indisputable; his genetic and agronomic innovations have produced wheat, corn, and rice yields that were inconceivable at the start of his work. As a result, many countries no longer need to import these commodities, prices have dropped, more people have access to these basic crops, and a significant number of people have improved nutrition. As table 1.1 shows, worldwide per capita consumption of calories, proteins, and lipids increased significantly from the middle of the 1960s to the end of the 1990s.

During the 1990s food stocks generally surpassed world demand by 20 percent. Today agricultural production is more than adequate to feed 6 billion human beings. Cereal production alone, at about 2 billion tonnes (330 kilograms per capita per year, or 3,600 calories per capita per day), could to a large extent meet the energy needs of the world's population if it were well distributed (Perry, 1990; Food and Agriculture Organization, 2000a). The problem of how to feed millions of people as world population in-

TABLE 1.1. Evolution of world food availability

Years	Calories Per capita/day	Protein	Fat
		Per capita/day (g)	
Average 1967–69	2,343	64.1	52.5
Average 1977–79	2,511	66.4	57.2
Average 1987–89	2,693	71.3	66.9
Average 1997–99	2,803	75.1	73.6
Increase (%)	19.6	17.2	40.2

Source: Food and Agriculture Organization, 2001a.

creased was solved, and fear of chronic food shortages for large parts of the world turned out to be unfounded. At the beginning of the new millennium the world's 5.8 billion people had on average 15 percent more food per person than did the 4 billion people who existed twenty years earlier. Still, millions of people do not get enough to eat. Between 1974 and 1996 the number of people estimated to be suffering from hunger and malnutrition increased from 450 to 800 million. This terrible situation can only be resolved if the economic aspects are addressed. Hunger and malnutrition are very closely associated with absolute poverty. More than 1 billion people, most of them living in rural areas, subsist on less than one U.S. dollar per day (Kashambuzi, 1999; Food and Agriculture Organization, 2000b; Bohnet, 2001).

In a time of unprecedented plenty, 826 million people still do not have enough to eat. The Food and Agriculture Organization's publication *The State of Food Insecurity in the World 2000* (2000b) states that little progress is being made in bringing about significant reductions in the number of hungry people in the world. Socioeconomic studies show increasingly unfavorable income prospects in undeveloped countries in which serious food shortages exist. This means a continuation of poverty and malnutrition in these locations for the foreseeable future (Food and Agriculture Organization, 1996, 2000a, 2001b).

The green revolution increased the production of crops in significant quantities sufficient to feed the world. This extraordinary effort, however, was not accompanied by another and equally important need: giving expanding populations the money to buy these crops. The result is that production has surpassed demand, but it does not meet the needs of the people.

TABLE I.2. Worldwide yield of the four main crops (corn, wheat, soybeans, and rice), 1961–63 and 1998–2000

Crop	1961–63	1998–2000	Increase %	1961–63	1998–2000	Increase %
	hg/ha			t/1,000 capita		
Corn	19,854	43,418	119	66.8	101	51.2
Wheat	11,423	27,168	138	74.9	97.8	30.6
Soybeans	11,411	22,182	94	8.7	26.7	206.2
Rice	19,388	38,623	99	73.1	99.6	36.3

Source: Food and Agriculture Organization, 2001a.

If we analyze the concept of Malthus, who said that the world's population will die of starvation, from the point of view of production, it seems to be in error. But if we view his concept from the standpoint of distribution, it becomes reality.

Genetic improvement and intensive use of fertilizers and agrochemicals along with widespread distribution of improved crop production techniques have increased production of the four main crops—wheat, corn, rice, and soybeans—in a dramatic way. Between the beginning of the 1960s and the end of the 1990s, yields of these crops increased 138, 119, 99, and 94 percent, respectively, while availability per capita increased 31, 51, 36, and 206 percent (table 1.2).

Many regions have benefited from the green revolution. There have been significant increases in yields in several countries, particularly with large-scale irrigated agriculture. Increased production arose not only because yields increased but also because crops could be planted in ecosystems previously considered as limited for cropping, thanks to newly developed varieties and technological packages. Thus, regions that imported a number of grains in the past are self-sufficient today, and some have even become exporters. In the case of rice, Indonesia, Thailand, and Vietnam are examples.

The green revolution also brought unwanted consequences to millions of growers. One of the more difficult problems that has appeared frequently in the history of agriculture is overproduction. When this occurs, prices drop. Falling agricultural prices are particularly disastrous to the agricultural sectors of undeveloped countries as there are no production subsidies to compensate for decreasing incomes. Overproduction affects all agricultural sectors, from very small to very large producers. For instance, in South

America the small cassava (*Manihot esculenta* C.) growers from Córdoba and Sucre, Colombia, cannot compete with cassava powder imported from Africa, and the huge wheat producers of the Humid Pampas in Argentina saw prices drop 53 percent in twelve years (Ayerza, 1996a). On an international level, over the last twenty years the prices of rice, corn, and wheat have decreased 50 percent or more (Agroenlínea, 2001). Globalization and overproduction are responsible for the reduced incomes of farmers throughout the world today. Even in regions that were heavily influenced by the green revolution, many small, poorly equipped, and very low income farmers have been unable to take advantage of new methods of production. Because they are unable to invest and progress, their incomes have fallen as a result of decreased agricultural prices, and many of them now live in extreme poverty, having been forced to leave their farms.

We can try to explain this problem a little better by quoting two paragraphs from the report entitled *The State of Food and Agriculture*:

Because of falling agricultural prices, the already low cash income of these farmers becomes insufficient to maintain and entirely renew their equipment and inputs and thus further erodes their production capacity. At this stage, an able-bodied member of the family can still be sent out to find temporary or permanent work elsewhere, although this weakens farm production capacity still further. The temporary survival of the farm only becomes possible by means of decapitalization (sale of livestock, non-renewal of equipment), under consumption, under nutrition and the migration of part of the workforce.

Increasingly poorly equipped and badly fed, these farmers are obligated to concentrate their efforts on short-term returns and to neglect the maintenance of the cultivated ecosystem. This neglect takes the form of poor maintenance of irrigation systems, slash-and-burn of ever younger fallow, insufficient weeding, sale of livestock and reduced transfer of fertility to the soil. The economic non-renewal of the productive system leads to non-renewal of fertility of the cultivated ecosystem. (Food and Agriculture Organization, 2000a:190)

In underdeveloped, agriculture-dominated countries the green revolution and globalization have caused the paradox of hunger and abundance. This arises because the demand for food in the marketplace is low, as the hungry people of the world have no buying capacity. This situation, which has taken place during the last decade in countries such as Argentina, Brazil, Mexico, and Peru, has been accentuated because of specialization, which in turn has reduced exportable products. Subsequently, as food imports increased, so did agricultural exports, worsening trade balances (Conway and Barbier, 1990; Mingione and Pugliese, 1994; Kashambuzi, 1999). Not only does this increase food dependence, it also changes dietary habits.

Agricultural overproduction and surplus crops are not simply numbers to be dealt with. Many people suffer with this reality every day, creating millions of stories charged with drama and misery. To know one story is the best way to understand the drama that exists today as millions of people suffer.

Rosa Huaman

This story, which is recent and sad, has never been written and has not even been completely told until now. It is the story of a Peruvian woman living in one of the terrible suburbs of the city of Ica, 300 kilometers south of Lima, the capital of Peru. These housing developments are pompously called "young towns," but in reality they are miserable slums. Living conditions are infinitely poorer than those of the *villas de emergencia* of Buenos Aires and even worse than the sadly famous *favelas* of Rio de Janeiro and the slums of Bombay and Calcutta. These suburbs don't have running water, electricity, garbage collection, paved roads, or sidewalks. Human excrement is piled everywhere and remains forever because it never, yes never, rains in Ica. This is terrible and impossible to visualize. The great majority of people who live along the Peruvian coast in cities such as Ica are born, live, and die surrounded by their garbage and their misery.

Rosa Huaman, the woman in this story, was not born in Ica. She came into the world more than 4,877 meters above sea level in the Peruvian altiplano, close to Lake Titicaca. There, on the island of the Sun and the Moon, according to the legend, two brothers, Manco Capac and Mama Ocllo, were born. They started the short-lived (lasting just one hundred years) but immortal Inca Empire.

Rosa was short, copper skinned, and sturdily built. She was a pure native. In her veins ran ancient Peruvian blood, as she was a descendant of the Quechua nation. Rosa and her family lived on what she could produce on her little piece of ancestral land, which had been overused and made almost desertlike by trying to force it to meet the basic needs of the family. In addition, frost and little rain also limited its production.

The imbalance between production and the needs of the family continued to grow, until the end for Rosa and her family became clear. Heavy rainfall from the phenomenon known as El Niño ruined the potato crop. Still, the family had some reserves of naturally dehydrated potatoes, made as their ancestors had made them even before the Incas. Subsequently, La Niña (the opposite of El Niño) arrived, bringing cold and drought. This destroyed the next potato crop and Rosa's hopes.

The chronic lack of work in the region, made more serious during the previous decade by political actions such as agrarian reform, the bloody attacks of the Shining Path (Maoist) guerrillas, and the barbarian acts of the government soldiers, made it impossible for many families to remain. So Rosa, like thousands of other Quechuas, Aymaras, and other natives, was forced to leave forever the land her family had inhabited.

Rosa took the few things she had, wrapped them in a blanket she had knitted from the fiber of her two llamas, put the blanket on her back, and bound a *lliclla* (a warmer and shorter blanket) on her chest with her youngest *guagua* (baby) inside. Then, with her three other children walking silently behind her, she started down the mountain, away from her beloved Andean land. Her husband, Hermilio, had started down the same road three years ago but had not been heard from since.

At the end of her trip an even harder lifestyle awaited her: how to survive in the slums that arise around the overpopulated coastal cities. The city of Ica was to be Rosa and her children's destiny. Ica was a destination without return, but Rosa did not know that, and in reality she had no other option. In the Andes there was nothing to prevent her and her children's hunger, and maybe Inti (the god of the sun in Inca mythology) would help her find her beloved Hermilio.

With some boards she built a "house" and survived by eating food from Ica's garbage dump. A short time after her arrival in September 1995 she was told that the potato harvest had started in a field surrounding Ica's airport. To get there she knew she would have to walk all night, but maybe, just maybe, she could obtain some potatoes that had been missed by the harvesting crew (in Peru potatoes are harvested by hand) or that had been discarded because of their small size or bad condition.

When she arrived at the field with her *guagua* on her back she was tired but happy. The harvest was not yet finished. Surrounding the 2-hectare field were more than one hundred people—men, women, and children—waiting, as was Rosa, for the same luck. This year, as happens cyclically, there was an overproduction of potatoes in other parts of the world, and Peru was importing them at a very low price. This situation was seriously harming Peru, as locally grown potatoes had to compete with the price of imported potatoes. Domestic potatoes were being sold so cheap that the growers could not pay their expenses. What a paradox!

A supervisor, looking both defiant and scared at the same time, with a gun hanging from his waist where everybody could see it, watched the silent crowd surrounding the field. He was not alone. Four guards with their rifles on their hips pointing to the sky were with him. They were constantly looking over the crowd as workers in the field harvested the potatoes. The atmosphere was tense but seemed under control. After all, the participants were just following the script set out by customs that had developed following the failure of the brutal agrarian reform of the 1960s.

Suddenly, something happened. With no word or gesture the silent group of observers surged into the field and started to pick what they could. The overseer and his collaborators intended to dissuade them first by yelling and then by firing their guns. Later they would say that they fired the shots into the air, that they never pointed their guns at the people. The truth is that Rosa fell down and died. Everything lasted just a few minutes. When the people ran from the field carrying their meager potato harvest, only the body of Rosa Huaman remained. Her *lojo* (black felt hat) and her *guagua* were no longer with her; someone had taken them.

That very night we ate with the general administrator of the farm, the one who had sown the potatoes. This was "an unfortunate episode," he assured us. "Everybody said it was an accident," he added in a very satisfied way. "Who was everybody?" we asked. There was no answer, just silence. No one was ever imprisoned for Rosa's death, and we never ate with the administrator again.

This sad story occurred in modern Peru, but unfortunately it is repeated in countless African, Latin American, and Asian countries. There are 826 million people at risk of dying of starvation. Rosa Huaman and her family are in that number.

This story points out the relationship between food production and food needs without considering the buying capacity of the thousands of Rosas living in our world. Agricultural production is increasing, but millions of farmers cannot add new technologies to increase their yields and maintain their incomes high enough to avoid abandoning their lands. The Food and Agriculture Organization (2000b) has determined that a large majority of the people who are chronically undernourished live in poor farming communities.

New Crops

When prices of traditional crops drop, the first areas to be abandoned are those regions considered marginal for production. Marginal areas are defined as having poor soil, climate, and/or infrastructure. Without doubt, regions that have low yields because of climatic problems, because they require the use of irrigation and high levels of fertilizer and agrochemicals, and/or because they are farthest from markets are the first to be abandoned. If growers do not have alternative crops to plant, they have no choice but to leave their land.

Overproduction of traditional crops and subsequent price drops are also causing problems in developed countries (United States Department of Agriculture, 1988, 1996; United Nations, 1990; Brown and Golding, 1992; Food and Agricultural Policy Research Institute, 1995). In the United States and the European Union overproduction of traditional crops has caused farmers to become increasingly dependent on subsidies. Subsidies are under increased pressure to be cut so as to reduce overproduction and the cost of farm support programs. The technologies that have produced higher yields are themselves being challenged by strong environmental lobbies, and there is concern over the limited number of crop species on which the world's population depends. Reliance on a small number of crops carries great agricultural and nutritional risks, as monocultures are extremely vulnerable to catastrophic failures brought about by disease or climate variations.

Close to 1.4 million living species have been identified. The major ones are 750,000 insects, 41,000 vertebrates, and 250,000 plants. The remainder are invertebrates, mushrooms, algae, and microorganisms (Wilson, 1988). Almost 3,000 plants have been investigated for food or other uses; however, just 100 have been studied in depth. Throughout time humans have tended to concentrate on obtaining nourishment from a few plants. Today, only 150 plant species are cultivated, twelve of them providing approximately 75 percent of our food. Four of them produce more than half of the food consumed. Most people in the world are fed with cereals such as wheat, rice, millet, and sorghum; tubers such as potatoes, sweet potatoes, and cassava; legumes such as beans, soybeans, and peanuts; and other crops such as sugarcane, sugar beets, cocoa, and bananas (National Research Council, 1975; Harlan, 1992).

In 1992 the general director of the Food and Agriculture Organization alerted the world to this backward evolution and said that as a result human nutrition was suffering. He also pointed out that the vulnerability of agriculture was increasing and that humans were in danger, as they had only a few sources from which to obtain food (Vietmeyer, 1978; Saouma, 1992). The human food supply now depends on a small number of species, and the failure of one of them could mean starvation for millions of people.

Medical, nutritional, and government recommendations emphasizing the need for nutritional diversity from a health standpoint have come at a time when humanity has restricted its diet to a few plant species. The need to return to searching for new plants to broaden available food types and hence diversify the human diet is urgent if we are to ensure the future of humanity. This can be done by bringing new crops into production and by increasing the production of underutilized crops.

It is time to consider rescuing a number of ancient crops that were forced into obscurity through the passage of time and with changes in culture and use. Cultural discrimination against some crops caused them to disappear, as did substitution of old crops with new ones for political-cultural reasons. Copying dominant models and replacing the uses and customs of many regions with those from others have diminished the variability in foods that previously existed. Since the beginning of time conquerors have imposed their systems on defeated nations, including the replacement of customs and nutritional habits.

The American continent was not an exception to this. After Christopher Columbus arrived many basic foods of the New World were replaced with crops brought by the Spanish conquerors. Thousands of acres under the control of the Aztec, Inca, and other cultures were planted with crops that were unknown to the conquerors. With the collapse of these cultures following the conquest, most of these crops fell into disuse. Many of the indigenous species possessed qualities equal or superior to those of the foreign ones, but this was disregarded during colonial times, when consumer demand in Europe largely dictated the cultivation and research priorities in the New World. Also, food preferences of local populations were so influenced by European food habits that in many places demand for native crops declined significantly (National Research Council, 1975; Vietmeyer, 1978). As a consequence, most pre-Columbian crops were retained only in isolated communities and today in many cases are endangered (National Research Council, 1989).

The need to diversify available food types provides an opportunity to save ancestral crops before they disappear and bring them back to their original importance. Adding other species will diversify agricultural production, improve diets, help prevent illnesses, and lower food costs as well as decrease the pressure on agricultural markets brought about by overproduction, increase growers' incomes and improve the quality of their lives, and prevent forced migration of people in undeveloped countries to the misery belts surrounding huge cities.

A good example of one of these forgotten pre-Columbian crops is chia (*Salvia hispanica* L.), one of the four main Aztec crops at the time of Columbus's arrival in the New World. Chia seed contains oil with the highest omega-3 fatty acid content available from plants. Today this species is practically unknown from a nutritional standpoint; instead, it is known only because of its use in Chia Pets. This book has been written to spread the knowledge of chia's nutritional aspects and to show how humans could benefit from making it a commercial crop.

TWO

The Importance of Omega-3 Fatty Acids

The Evolution of Our Diet

In the beginning men and women lived by eating what they collected, fished, or hunted from their natural habitat. Later they lived by consuming what they grew or raised. Today most people consume what others produce. The land has not lost its essentiality as the basis to sustain people, but the relationship has become so distant that most people do not know anything about agriculture and its importance to mankind.

A recent survey in the United States demonstrated this reality when some people were asked if they knew where their food originated. Some of them answered, "In supermarkets." For those people words such as overgrazing, saltification, desertification, drought, and others related to food production do not have any meaning. This state of affairs is closely associated with the dramatic decrease in the number of people directly involved with agriculture. As was the case with many countries at that time, the United States in 1900 was predominantly rural, with nearly 40 percent of the population living on farms. By the 1990s only 1.9 percent of Americans were living in farm households (Beale, 2001).

With human evolution, changes in living were accompanied by changes in food. Modern diets are very different from those of closely related primates and almost certainly from those of early hominids and preagricultural but anatomically modern humans who lived 30,000 years ago (Wadley and Martin, 1993). Humans have been on earth for 3–5 million years, and for more than 99 percent of this time they lived as hunters and gatherers. Only in the last 10,000 years, from the Neolithic to the present, did they domesticate plants and animals and transition to an agricultural lifestyle (Engel, 1987; Harlan, 1992). It has been estimated that the typical diet of the Paleolithic period (2 million—10,000 B.C.) consisted of 50 percent plant-based foods and 50 percent from animal origin. Preagricultural foods came from wild game—such as deer, bison, horses, mammoths—fish, wild plants, whole grains, and honey, but no dairy products, oils, and salt were consumed (Cowan and Watson, 1992; Lichtenstein, 1999).

According to Simopoulos (1999a), the spontaneous mutation rate for DNA is estimated at 0.5 percent per million years. Therefore, during the agricultural period there has been little if any change in human DNA. Most human evolution took place during the time of Paleolithic diets; hence, genetically, humans remain adapted to a Paleolithic diet (Wadley and Martin, 1993; Eaton and Eaton III, 1999, 2000). Data from archaeological findings support the concept that the genetic makeup of human beings as it exists today was developed by a Paleolithic diet. Epidemiological studies and controlled experiments strongly support the need to return to that diet (Eaton et al., 1998; Simopoulos, 1998; Eaton and Eaton III, 2000).

Major changes in the human food supply and energy expenditure first took place during the agricultural period and then again during the Industrial Revolution (Simopoulos, 1998; Lichtenstein, 1999). Modern Western diets (those prevailing in Europe and the United States today) are characterized by increased amounts of fat, saturated fat, trans-fatty acids, and omega-6 fatty acids and decreased amounts of omega-3 fatty acids. The ratio of omega-6 to omega-3 fatty acids is now between 10:1 and 20:1, whereas during the Paleolithic period it was 1:1 (Eaton et al., 1998). Table 2.1 compares modern Western diets with a Paleolithic diet.

Differences between Paleolithic and Western diets have arisen not only as a result of changes in nutritional habits but also because of changes in food composition. The first change occurred during the agricultural revolution, when consumption of animal products decreased and plant product consumption increased to 90 percent of the diet in some cases (Eaton et al., 1996). Today animal products have once again reached significant levels in

TABLE 2.1. Characteristics of Paleolithic and modern Western diets

Nutrient	Paleolithic diet	Modern Western diet
Energy	moderate	high
Protein	high	low—moderate
Animal	high	low—moderate
Vegetable	very low	low—moderate
Carbohydrate	low—moderate	moderate
Fiber	high	low
Fat	low	high
Animal	low	high
Vegetable	very low	moderate—high
Omega-6:omega-3 fatty acid ratio	low (2:4)	high (12:0)
Vitamins (mg/day)		
Ascorbate	604	93
Folate	0.36	0.18
Riboflavin	6.49	1.71
Thiamin	3.91	1.42
Vitamin A	17.2	7.8
Vitamin E	32.8	8.5

Sources: Simopoulos, 1998a; Eaton and Eaton III, 2000.

the diet (Garn and Leónard, 1989; Eaton, Eaton III, and Konner, 1997). The second change occurred during the Industrial Revolution, when food composition changed because of food fractioning and processing.

According to Dr. Artemis Simopoulos, president of the Center for Genetics, Nutrition and Health in Washington, D.C., the diets of North American and other Western countries have changed radically over the past 100–150 years. Speaking at the Flax Council of Canada conference held in Winnipeg on 3 December 1996, Simopoulos said: "The rapid dietary change over this short period of time is a totally new phenomenon in human history" (Flax Council of Canada, 1996).

Table 2.2 compares the macronutrient intakes of Paleolithic humans to current Western diets. Leaf and Weber (1987) estimated average daily intake for late Paleolithic humans at 3,000 calories, with the diet comprised of 35 percent animal products and 65 percent vegetable products. In spite of the high intake of animal products, late Paleolithic diets were lower in total fat and higher in polyunsaturated fatty acids than current Western diets. According to Leaf and Weber (1987), this difference arises because game animals were lean, and since they foraged for their food rather than being fattened with grains, as is done with domesticated meat sources, little of

TABLE 2.2. Daily macronutrient intake for late Paleolithic
and current Western diets

	Intake	
Nutrient	Paleolithic	Current Western
Protein (g)	251	90
Animal	191	62
Vegetable	60	28
Fat (g)	71	142
Animal	30	82
Vegetable	41	60
PUFA:SAT ratio[1]	1.4	0.44
Cholesterol (mg)	591	600
Carbohydrate (g)	334	335
Fiber (g)	46	20

Sources: Modified from Eaton and Konner, 1985; Leaf and Weber, 1987.
1. PUFA: polyunsaturated fatty acid; SAT: saturated fatty acid.

their fat was saturated, as the plants they consumed contained relatively high percentages of polyunsaturated fatty acids. Eaton and Konner (1985) noted that the fats of wild animals contain appreciable amounts of omega-3 fatty acids. Because the vegetable portion of Paleolithic diets also contained appreciable amounts of omega-3 fatty acids, it seems likely that these diets contained significant amounts of omega-3 fatty acids. It would appear that the omega-3 fatty acids were mainly alpha-linolenic acid, with only low quantities of long-chain omega-3 fatty acids such as docosahexaenoic acid (DHA) consumed (Eaton and Eaton III, 1999).

Animal domestication brought about a change in food consumption and composition, especially in terms of omega-3 and omega-6 fatty acid content. Domesticated animals have higher total fat and saturated fatty acid contents, decreased omega-3 and omega-6 fatty acid levels, and higher omega-6 to omega-3 ratios than do wild animals. With the arrival of the Industrial Revolution animal food changed from grass, which provided a balanced omega-6 to omega-3 fatty acid ratio, to grain, which is high in omega-6 and low in omega-3 fatty acids. Compositional changes took place with chicken, pork, eggs, and milk as well. This also was the case with aquaculture, as fish went from eating seaweed, which is high in omega-3 fatty acids, to eating grains similar to those fed to domestic animals (Eaton et al., 1998; Simopoulos, 1998; Cordain, 1999; Lichtenstein, 1999).

People have become very dependent upon cereal grains. Hunter-gatherers ate more than one hundred species of plants and animals in the course of a year. Modern humans depend on barely twenty species of plants, four mammals (cattle, sheep, pigs, and goats), and one bird (chicken) for the bulk of their nourishment. From the twenty plant species eaten, only four are cereals (wheat, corn, rice, and barley), and these form 70 percent of modern Western diets. This dependence on a few species puts Western civilizations in a very precarious situation if diseases or pests were to threaten any of these plants (Solbrig and Solbrig, 1990; Harlan, 1992; Cordain, 1999). Additionally, intensive medical and nutritional research has demonstrated the importance a diversified diet has in maintaining human health (Krauss et al., 2000).

Although heart diseases are some of the major diseases in which diet plays an important role, others that strike many people today such as depression, breast cancer, lung cancer, colorectal cancer, and stomach cancer are also affected by diet (Okuyama, Kobayashi, and Watanabe, 1997; Wu and Meydani, 1998; Rose and Connolly, 2000). In the United States four of the ten leading causes of death have strong links to diet and annually cost over $200 billion in treatment and lost productivity (Economic Research Service, 2001).

Scientific evidence has shown that cereal grains have significant nutritional shortcomings, and differences between genetic dietary needs and the human diet are responsible for many chronic diseases (Eaton et al., 1998; Cordain, 1999). One of many examples is found in the Tohono O'odham nation in Arizona. It has the highest rate of diabetes in the world; more than 50 percent of the adult population is affected. Today these people eat a typical Western diet. When native plants that were an integral part of their diet are reintroduced into their diet, positive changes take place. Blood sugar levels slowly rise, and there is a low insulin response (Nabhan, 1989; Balick and Cox, 1997).

The main deficiencies in cereals are vitamin A, vitamin C, beta-carotene, calcium, sodium, omega-3 fatty acids, and amino acids such as lysine and threonine. Another problem is that cereals possess a significant imbalance between omega-3 and omega-6 fatty acids, favoring the latter. When these cereals are combined with an increased use of vegetable oils, which have equal or poorer ratios, they form a diet that is very different from that recommended by health agencies.

The Diets of Pre-Columbian Mesoamerican Descendants Living in the United States

A number of authors have reported on the wide varieties of food eaten by ancient American nations. Before Columbus's arrival, even the lowest social groups ate nutritionally more balanced and healthier foods than the people of Mexico and Peru eat today (Ortiz de Montellano, 1978; Antunez de Mayolo, 1981; Engel, 1987). When the Spaniards arrived in America, the Aztec diet included up to 229 different plants (Sahagún, 1579). The Seri, Tarahumara, and Huasteco nations in Mexico still hold to tradition and eat highly diversified diets, consuming 94, 137, and 201 native species, respectively (Felger and Moser, 1985; Hernández-Bermejo and León, 1992).

Although in the United States the word *Hispanic* embraces all people originating from Spanish-speaking countries, the largest percentage comes from Mexico and Central America, followed by South America. These people descended from the Aztec-Nahua, Maya, and Inca Empires, respectively. Aldrich and Variyam (2000) showed that the U.S. Hispanic population has health and mortality records that in many aspects are more favorable than those of the general U.S. population. According to the Centers for Disease Control and Prevention of the United States Department of Health and Human Services (1999), the U.S. Hispanic population has a significantly lower rate of death from cardiovascular diseases, coronary heart disease, stroke, and cancer than the general U.S. population and other major ethnicities.

Despite economic and educational disadvantages, people of Hispanic origin eat healthier diets than do non-Hispanic whites. This includes eating 11 percent less dietary fat and saturated fatty acids (United States Department of Agriculture, 2000). Their traditional eating patterns, however, change dramatically in just one generation in the United States. A study conducted by Sylvia Guedelman and Barbara Abrams at the University of California at Berkeley that is cited by Aldrich and Variyam (2000) compared the dietary quality of Mexican immigrants to second-generation Mexican Americans and non-Hispanic whites. They concluded that as people of Mexican origin moved from the first to the second generation, the quality of their diet deteriorated and approximated that of white non-Hispanics.

Aldrich and Variyam (2000) reported decreased dietary quality with Hispanic English speakers compared to Hispanic Spanish speakers. People of Hispanic origin who do not speak English have a nutritional diet much closer to the recommendations made by the U.S. government in the dietary guidelines for Americans and the food guide pyramid than do those who speak English. Cultural integration, which is often accompanied by an improved economic situation, erodes quality of diet. This suggests that for non-English-speaking Hispanics an ancestral origin is behind their eating habits (United States Department of Agriculture, 1997; Variyam, 1999).

Animal Fats and Vegetable Oils in Human Diets

Oil crops, their products, and their byproducts constitute the second most valuable commodity in the world. Between 1996 and 1999 worldwide lipid production was 117.2 million tons. Of this, 78.5 million tons were used in human nutrition (table 2.3): 59.6 million tons of vegetable oils and 18.9 million tons of animal fat (Food and Agriculture Organization, 2001). In the last forty years worldwide consumption of lipids has increased at a rate of almost 3.2 million tons per year (Food and Agriculture Organization, 2001). It is interesting to note that in most of the world dietary oil consumption is closely related to buying power (Downey, Robbelen, and Ashri, 1989; Berger, 1989). At the beginning of the 1960s vegetable oils comprised 55.1 percent of the total lipidic diet, while today they comprise more than 75 percent of the diet (table 2.3). Although the global tendency is increasing consumption of vegetable oils and decreasing consumption of animal fats, this is really only taking place in developed countries. In undeveloped countries animal fat intake has not decreased; instead, it has significantly increased.

Of the vegetable oils used in human nutrition, 99 percent come from a dozen sources (soybean, sunflower, corn, cottonseed, sesame, rice, palm, copra, palm kernel, peanut, canola, and olive), with 80 percent coming from only five crops (soybean, peanut, sunflower, canola, and palm). All of these oils are low or very low in omega-3 fatty acid content and have high to medium quantities of omega-6 fatty acids (table 2.4). Consumption of these oils causes an imbalance in the omega-6 and omega-3 fatty acid ratio in the diet and is manifested in the dramatic increase in chronic diseases that

TABLE 2.3. Quantity of lipids (fats) used in human food, 1961–63 and 1996–99

Region	1961–63[1] Total tons[2]	kg/capita	1996–99[1] Total tons[2]	kg/capita	Increment (%) Total tons	kg/capita
World						
Total lipids	27.9	8.9	78.5	13.4	181.4	50.6
Vegetable oils	15.4	4.9	59.6	10.2	287	108.2
Animal fats	12.5	4	18.9	3.2	51.2	−20
Developed countries						
Total lipids	18.9	19	32.4	24.9	71.4	31.1
Vegetable oils	8.4	8.5	21.4	16.4	154.8	92.9
Animal fats	10.5	10.5	11	8.5	4.8	−19
Developing countries						
Total lipids	8.8	4.1	46	10.1	422.7	146.3
Vegetable oils	6.8	3.2	38.2	8.4	461.8	162.5
Animal fats	2	0.9	7.8	1.7	290	88.9

Source: Food and Agriculture Organization, 2001a.
1. Average per year.
2. 1,000 metric tons.

have occurred in the second half of the twentieth century (Okuyama, Kobayashi, and Watanabe, 1997; British Nutrition Foundation, 1999; Simopoulos, 1999a).

Lipids, Fatty Acids, and Human Nutrition

Lipids and their role in human nutrition is one of the most important areas in nutrition research (Food and Agriculture Organization, 1994; Okuyama, Kobayashi, and Watanabe, 1997). From an energetic point of view, lipids are more important than proteins and carbohydrates. Lipids contain 9 calories per gram, compared to proteins and carbohydrates, which have only 4 calories (Garrison and Somer, 1990; United States Department of Agriculture and United States Department of Health and Human Services, 1995).

Dietary lipids are comprised mainly of triglycerides and small amounts of phospholipids, cholesterol, and other sterols. Triglycerides are the main form in which lipids are stored in the body. Chemically, triglycerides are glycerol molecules esterified (converted into an ester) with three fatty acids. The position of each fatty acid in the molecular structure determines whether the triglycerides are absorbed as 2-monoglycerides or as free fatty

TABLE 2.4. Relative amounts of fatty acids in vegetable oils (percent)

Crop	Saturated	Oleic	Linoleic	Linolenic	Other
Babassu	83.1	15.1	1.7	0	0.1
Canola	6	64.1	18.7	9.2	2
Castor	2	5	4	0.5	88.5
Chia	9.4	7.8	20.2	62.7	0
Coconut	91.4	6.5	1.5	0	0.5
Corn	14.5	27.5	57	0.9	0.1
Cottonseed	28.6	17.6	53.3	0.3	0.1
Flaxseed	9.4	19.9	15.9	52.7	2
Jojoba	0	12	0	0	88
Oleic corn	11.3	64.5	22.1	0.6	1.5
Oleic safflower	7.9	79.7	12	0.2	0.2
Oleic sunflower	8	87	5	0	0
Olive	17.4	71.1	10	0.6	0.9
Palm kernel	83.9	13.7	2	0	0.1
Peanut	51.3	38.8	9.4	0.3	0.2
Rapeseed	4.4	23.8	14.6	7.3	49.9
Safflower	9	13.1	77.7	0	0.2
Sesame	15.6	41.2	43	0.2	0
Soybean	15.2	23.4	53.2	7.8	0.4
Sunflower	12.3	18.6	68.2	0.5	0.4

acids, thus influencing fatty acid availability. A number of fatty acids can be present in the same fat, and identical fatty acids can be found in various fats. The physical properties of lipids are strongly influenced by the nature of the constituent fatty acids (Chow, 1992a; Kelly, 1999).

Fatty acids are the building blocks from which other lipids are made in the body. All fatty acids are comprised of a chain of carbon atoms to which are attached hydrogen atoms, forming a hydrocarbon chain. Fatty acids are classified as short chain (fewer than six carbons), medium chain (six to ten carbons), or long chain (twelve or more carbons). More than 90 percent of all fatty acids have an even number of carbon atoms. Fatty acids are also classified as saturated (lacking double bonds), monounsaturated (containing a single double bond), or polyunsaturated (containing more than one double bond) (figure 2.1). Polyunsaturated fatty acids are subdivided into those whose first double bond occurs either three carbon atoms from the methyl carbon (omega-3 or n-3) or six carbon atoms from the methyl carbon (omega-6 or n-6) (figure 2.1) (Lobb, 1992; Katan, 1990; Naudet, 1996; Kelly, 1999).

Fatty acids stimulate and maintain life functions in humans and are con-

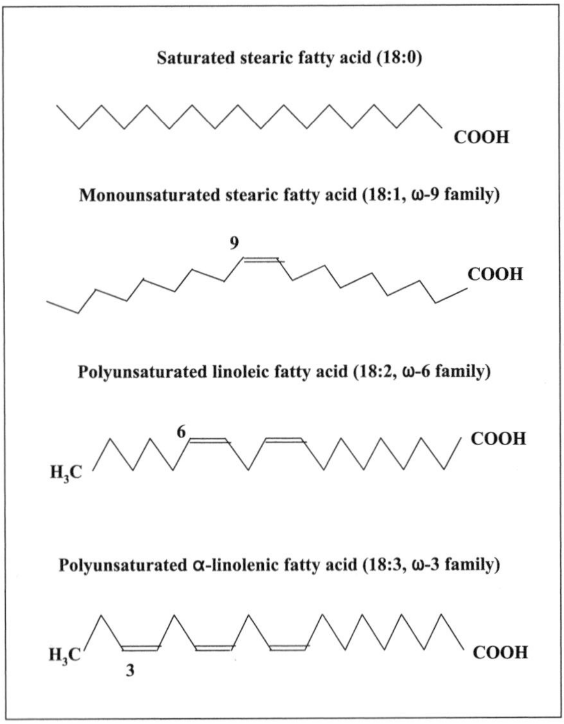

FIGURE 2.1.

Basic structure of fatty acids.

Saturated stearic fatty acid (18:0)

COOH

Monounsaturated stearic fatty acid (18:1, ω-9 family)

9

COOH

Polyunsaturated linoleic fatty acid (18:2, ω-6 family)

6

COOH

H₃C

Polyunsaturated α-linolenic fatty acid (18:3, ω-3 family)

H₃C

3

COOH

sidered a macronutrient in human nutrition. In Western diets (Europe, the United States, and Canada) fatty acids generally constitute the major source of calories. On the other hand, in Asia and undeveloped countries carbohydrates provide the main caloric resource (Nelson, 1992).

Fatty acids and their metabolic products serve three basic functions:

1. They act as a highly efficient energy reserve that provides protection against external agents like cold weather (Muggli and Clough, 1994; Nettleton, 1995).
2. They are a fundamental constituent of cellular membranes, giving them an elastic cover that protects each cell (Muggli and Clough, 1994; Nettleton, 1995).
3. They act as precursors (i.e., they are the source) from which are made an important group of hormonal compounds called prostaglandins, thromboxanes, and leukotrienes, which are involved in many physiological processes associated with the central nervous system, hormonal func-

tions, regulation of blood pressure, cholesterol transport, immunological mechanisms, and inflammatory reactions (American Heart Association, 1988; Welch and Borlakoglu, 1992; Muggli and Clough, 1994; Nettleton, 1995).

Saturated and monounsaturated fatty acids can be synthesized by the human body, while omega-3 and omega-6 polyunsaturated fatty acids cannot. Thus, the latter two polyunsaturated fatty acids must be provided by the diet and hence are classified as "essential fatty acids," while the former two are "nonessential fatty acids." Commonly, fatty acids are known by their initials: SFAs (saturated fatty acids), MUFAs (monounsaturated fatty acids), and PUFAs (polyunsaturated fatty acids) (Bjerve, Mostad, and Thorensen, 1987; Budowski, 1988; Bruckner, 1992; Welch and Borlakoglu, 1992; Muggli and Clough, 1994).

A deficiency in PUFAs in the diet is characterized by skin damage, excessive loss of water through the skin, and disturbances in growth and hormonal balance (Welch and Borlakoglu, 1992; Muggli and Clough, 1994; Nettleton, 1995). Omega-3 and omega-6 PUFAs have different physiological functions in the body (von Wullerstorff, 1990). The main omega-6 fatty acid is linoleic. In the body it can be metabolized into gamma-linolenic acid (GLA) and arachidonic acid (AA). The main omega-3 fatty acid is alpha-linolenic acid. Its metabolites are eicosapentaenoic acid (EPA) and docosahexaenoic acid (DHA) (Aveldaño, 1992; Mantzioris et al., 1995; Okuyama, Kobayashi, and Watanabe, 1997).

The transformation of linoleic acid into GLA and AA and alpha-linolenic acid into EPA and DHA in the body arises because of two processes, desaturation and elongation, that occur through the action of dasaturase and elongase enzymes (figure 2.2). As these two families of PUFAs share the same pathway for these processes, they compete for the same enzymes in the elongation and desaturation processes. Thus, under some conditions this presents a problem, as will be seen later in this chapter.

Lipids, Fatty Acids, and Coronary Heart Disease

Cardiovascular diseases account for about 1.4 million deaths (about 40 percent of total deaths) annually in the United States, making them the number

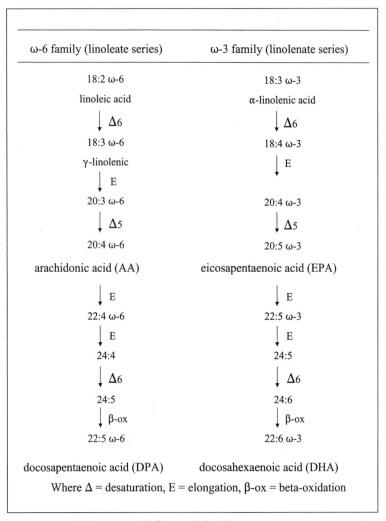

ω-6 family (linoleate series)	ω-3 family (linolenate series)
18:2 ω-6	18:3 ω-3
linoleic acid	α-linolenic acid
↓ Δ6	↓ Δ6
18:3 ω-6	18:4 ω-3
γ-linolenic	
↓ E	↓ E
20:3 ω-6	20:4 ω-3
↓ Δ5	↓ Δ5
20:4 ω-6	20:5 ω-3
arachidonic acid (AA)	eicosapentaenoic acid (EPA)
↓ E	↓ E
22:4 ω-6	22:5 ω-3
↓ E	↓ E
24:4	24:5
↓ Δ6	↓ Δ6
24:5	24:6
↓ β-ox	↓ β-ox
22:5 ω-6	22:6 ω-3
docosapentaenoic acid (DPA)	docosahexaenoic acid (DHA)

Where Δ = desaturation, E = elongation, β-ox = beta-oxidation

FIGURE 2.2. Polyunsaturated fatty acid families.

one cause of death in the country. (Cardiovascular diseases include rheumatic fever/rheumatic heart disease, hypertensive disease, ischemic [coronary] heart disease, diseases of pulmonary circulation, other forms of heart disease, cerebrovascular disease [stroke], vein diseases, and lymphatic and other diseases of the circulatory system. Depending upon availability, data for congenital cardiovascular anomalies are also included. (See the 2001 heart and stroke statistical update, glossary section, of the American Heart Association, www.americanheart.org) Coronary heart disease (CHD) accounts for about 681,000 deaths annually (American Heart Association, 2003a). (CHD includes acute myocardial infarction, other acute and subacute forms of ischemic [coronary] heart disease, old myocardial infarction, angina pectoris, and other forms of chronic ischemic heart disease.) CHD is related to nutrition and is a major concern in the United States and other Western countries (Schaefer et al., 1995; American Heart Association, 1988, 2001; British Nutrition Foundation, 1992).

The impact of CHD on Americans is not just confined to fatal cases. Survivors are mainly men between forty and forty-five years old. The decline in work capacity of this group due to CHD is a huge social and economic loss (Garrison and Somer, 1990). In 2003 the estimated indirect and direct cost of CHD in the United States was $130 billion and $352 billion, respectively, for all cardiovascular diseases. These figures include health expenditures as well as lost productivity (American Heart Association, 2003a).

CHD is a major health problem in many nations and is not exclusively a problem in developed countries (Nakajima, 1996; World Health Organization, 1995). In 1995 15 million people in the world died because of CHD. In Argentina, for instance, about 360,000 people per year, or 1 percent of the total population, are added to the list of patients with CHD. Of these, 23 percent die by sudden death, 42 percent suffer an acute infarct (a type of heart attack), 38 percent suffer progressive chest pain, and 7 percent have chest angina (a type of heart disease) (Alvarez, 1995).

CHD arises because of atherosclerosis, which is characterized by the deposition of fatty substances such as cholesterol and other lipids in the artery walls, thickening them. This process gradually reduces the diameter of the arteries and restricts blood flow. Inadequate blood flow may cause injury to or the death of tissue beyond the site of the reduced flow. In coronary arteries this leads to myocardial infarction (the death of part of the heart) or sudden death (American Heart Association, 1991).

Epidemiological as well as controlled experiments have demonstrated a direct relationship between CHD and diet. Extensive scientific evidence strongly supports a relationship between dietary cholesterol and saturated fatty acid intake and CHD (American Heart Association, 1990, 1991; Steinberg and Gotto, 1999; World Health Organization, 2003).

Risk Factors

During the last thirty years science has contributed enormously to the knowledge of the risk factors associated with CHD (American Heart Association, 1990; Chavali and Forse, 1994). The most important are high plasmatic cholesterol, smoking, high blood pressure, obesity, diabetes, high plasmatic triglycerides, sedentarism, high homocysteine levels, and family history (Hennekens, Buring, and Mayrent, 1990; Illingworth and Ullmann, 1990; Bruckner, 1992). The risk of suffering CHD is six times greater if an individual has three of these factors compared to having only one (Garrison and Somer, 1990).

The three major risk factors for CHD are smoking, high blood pressure, and high plasmatic cholesterol (Hennekens, Buring, and Mayrent, 1990). Smokers have a 60–80 percent greater risk of suffering CHD than do nonsmokers (Hennekens and Buring, 1985). People who have moderate blood pressure have approximately 40 percent less risk of suffering blockage (mortal or nonmortal) compared to people with high blood pressure. With a reduction in diastolic pressure of 8 millimeters, individuals have a 12 percent lower risk of suffering CHD (Hebert et al., 1988). When people with hypercholesterolemia reduce their cholesterol by 10 percent, they have 12 percent less risk of dying from a heart attack, 30 percent less risk of suffering a nonfatal heart attack, and 20 percent less risk of experiencing a first cardiac event (Consensus Conference, 1985; Smith et al., 1992). Other studies have shown that the decreases could be even larger (McDougall et al., 1995).

Cholesterol

The risk factor that has received the most attention in terms of its influence on CHD is cholesterol (Bruckner, 1992). It is well established that the risk of developing CHD is directly related to serum cholesterol levels. A study conducted in seven countries (the United States, Finland, Holland, Italy, Greece, Croatia-Serbia, and Japan) that used 12,467 subjects showed that even within different cultures cholesterol was directly related to mortality from CHD.

Four of the five major plasma lipoproteins have an important role in the transport of cholesterol and other lipids. Three of them have been associated with increased risk of CHD: very low density lipoprotein (VLDL), low-density lipoprotein (LDL), and intermediate-density lipoprotein (IDL). The last two are considered highly atherogenic (producing degenerative changes in arterial walls), with the atherogenicity of VLDL still being debated. This is opposite to high-density lipoprotein (HDL), which is anti-atherogenic. Epidemiological, clinical, and laboratory research has shown that increased quantities of LDL and IDL mean increased risk of CHD (American Heart Association, 1990; Berkow and Fletcher, 1992; Griffin, 1999; Steinberg and Gotto, 1999).

More than 100 million American adults have blood cholesterol levels greater than 200 milligrams/deciliter, while more than 40 million have levels of 240 milligrams/deciliter or greater. In adults, total cholesterol levels of 240 milligrams/deciliter or higher are considered high risk; levels from 200 to 239 milligrams/deciliter are considered borderline high risk (American Heart Association, 2001). Increased risk of CHD corresponds to increased cholesterol levels (Verschuren et al., 1995). Numerous investigations have shown that a decline in plasmatic cholesterol decreases or reverses the progression of cardiovascular diseases and can reduce CHD. Even in CHD high risk groups, the mortality index decreases with treatments that reduce plasmatic cholesterol (Berkow and Fletcher, 1992; Smith et al., 1992; Smith, Song, and Sheldon, 1993; McDougall et al., 1995).

A close relationship between high blood cholesterol and quantities of cholesterol, SFAs, and total fat consumed has been established (Keys, Anderson, and Grande, 1965; Ershow, Nocolosi, and Hayes, 1981; Schaefer et al., 1995). Also, as fat and edible oil composition varies, so do lipid concentrations in the plasma (Mensink and Katan, 1992; Jones, Toy, and Cha, 1994; Katan, Zock, and Mensink, 1995; Al et al., 1995).

Saturated Fatty Acids

According to the *Report of the Dietary Guidelines Advisory Committee on the Dietary Guidelines for Americans, 2000* (United States Department of Agriculture, 2000), SFAs have been identified as the predominant dietary factor contributing to CHD. This has been substantiated by an enormous number of studies in animal research, epidemiology, and metabolism as well as in clinical trials. Saturated fat is the principal dietary determinant of LDL cholesterol levels (Krauss et al., 2000). There is strong evidence that shows a close relationship between SFAs in the diet and the risk of suffering CHD

(American Heart Association, 1990, 1991; Katan, Zock, and Mensink, 1995; Choudhury, Tan, and Truswell, 1995). Early research generalized that consumption of foods high in saturated fats increased blood plasma cholesterol (Hegsted et al., 1965; Keys, Anderson, and Grande, 1965). Later work, however, showed that not all SFAs increase cholesterol to the same degree (Denke and Grundy, 1992; Temme, Mensink, and Hornstra, 1994).

The greatest effort to highlight the effects various SFAs have on health has been oriented toward palmitic fatty acid, of which palm oil contains 45.1 percent (White, 1992). More than one hundred studies on palmitic fatty acid have been directed and financed by the Malaysian government. In Malaysia palm oil represents between 7 and 8 percent of the gross domestic production of the country and provides about 300,000 jobs (Hashim, 1996). Malaysian studies on humans and laboratory animals have reported palm oil to give less pronounced effects on CHD than coconut oil, which is rich in lauric and myristic fatty acids (Ng et al., 1991; Choudhury, Tan, and Truswell, 1995). Some studies have even shown that palm oil is neutral in terms of cholesterol production while increasing HDL and decreasing LDL levels (Berger, 1996). These works contradict other studies that have shown palmitic fatty acid to increase LDL levels. Stearic acid, according to some research, has less capacity to increase blood cholesterol than do lauric, myristic, and palmitic acids (Katan, Zock, and Mensink, 1995; Nelson, 1992; Hassel, Mensing, and Gallaher, 1997). Thus, many scientists consider palm oil to be like other SFAs; that is, a high percentage in the diet will increase blood cholesterol (Katan, Zock, and Mensink, 1995).

The energy level of U.S. diets provided by lipids averages 38 percent, with 15 percent coming from SFAs. Nutritional recommendations state that total lipid calories should not be more than 30 percent, with SFAs being no more than 10 percent (American Heart Association, 1991; Taraszewaski and Jensen, 1994; United States Department of Agriculture and United States Department of Health and Human Services, 1995). The World Health Organization recommends a maximum of 10 percent of total lipid calories to come from SFAs but differs from the United States in that it sets the minimum at zero, because there is no specific requirement for SFAs in the human body (British Nutrition Foundation, 1992; World Health Organization, 2003). In Canada the Health and Welfare Department has recommended that energy provided by lipids not be more than 30 percent of the total, with energy from SFAs not being greater than 10 percent of total energy consumption (Zlotkin, 1996).

Monounsaturated Fatty Acids

Oleic acid is the most common MUFA (Nettleton, 1995) and is classified as nonessential because it can be synthesized in the human body (Muggli and Clough, 1994). The most common sources of oleic fatty acid are canola, olive, and sesame oil (table 2.4). The increasing commercial availability of oleic sunflower, which appeared at the end of the 1980s, and, more recently, oleic safflower and oleic corn has increased the use of this fatty acid worldwide (Williams, 1996; Floratech, 1996; Fick, 1988; White, 1992).

Oleic fatty acid, the common energy source of the Mediterranean diet provided through olive oil, has frequently been cited as having favorable effects on blood cholesterol. The advantages that the inhabitants of Crete exhibited regarding reduced CHD compared with Western contemporary societies, together with the determination that SFAs increase blood cholesterol, led to the generalization that the replacement of SFAs with MUFAs through the consumption of olive oil decreases cholesterol. Various investigations, however, differ notably on the effects that oleic acid has on blood cholesterol (Schaefer et al., 1995). The first published works showed oleic acid to have no effect (Hegsted et al., 1965; Keys, Anderson, and Grande, 1965). Later works determined that replacing SFAs with MUFAs did not bring additional benefits to those produced by PUFAs (Mensink and Katan, 1992; Mattson and Grundy, 1985). Herein a controversy arises, because it was not determined if the decrease in cholesterol happened because of the action of the MUFAs or was due to decreased SFA intake (Bruckner, 1992).

Decreased LDL and unchanged HDL levels were found when diets rich in SFAs were replaced by diets rich in oleic acid (Mattson and Grundy, 1985; Grundy, 1986; Katan, Zock, and Mensink, 1995). This information, however, comes from research in which safflower and oleic sunflower were used as the sources of oleic acid instead of olive oil (Liepa and Gorman, 1991). The use of these two sources of oleic fatty acid instead of olive oil introduces at least two other important variables. First, oils from safflower and oleic sunflower contain oleic acid plus a higher percentage of PUFAs, 78 and 14 percent, respectively, compared with only 8 percent in olive oil (Nettleton,

1995). Second, safflower and oleic sunflower have only 9 and 8 percent, respectively, SFA content (Floratech, 1996) compared to 14.9 percent for olive oil. These differences in fatty acid composition, combined with the differing effects that PUFAs and SFAs have on plasmatic cholesterol, could mask the effects observed.

Pedersen et al. (2000) reported that olive oil—rich diets result in higher concentrations of LDL cholesterol and LDL subfraction particles than do rapeseed and sunflower oil diets. The authors suggest that rapeseed and sunflower oil diets have more favorable effects on plasma lipid and lipoprotein concentrations in healthy subjects than does an olive oil diet. Other research looking into the processes that alter heart rhythm found they could not be controlled by substituting SFAs with oleic acid delivered through olive oil (McLennan, 1993; McLennan and Dallimore, 1994). These processes could be controlled by including safflower oil, probably not because of the oleic acid (64 percent) but rather because of the alpha-linolenic acid (9 percent) it contains (McLennan and Dallimore, 1994). Analysis of the available information leads one to conclude that the beneficial effects of oleic acid in general and olive oil in particular in terms of their effects on CHD were, at best, exaggerated (Renaud et al., 1995; James, 1995; Siguel, 1996; Pedersen et al., 2000).

Polyunsaturated Fatty Acids

Omega-3 Fatty Acids. During the last two decades of the twentieth century there was an explosion of research aimed at determining the relationship between omega-3 fatty acids and human health (Simopoulos, 1998; Li et al., 1999; Mantzioris et al., 2000). There is growing evidence that foods rich in omega-3 fatty acids, including alpha-linolenic acid and its metabolites, EPA and DHA, provide cardioprotective effects beyond those that can be attributed to improvement in blood lipoprotein profiles. The predominant beneficial effects include a reduction in sudden death, decreased risk of arrhythmia, lower plasma triglyceride levels, and reduced blood-clotting tendency (Okuyama, Kobayashi, and Watanabe, 1997; British Nutrition Foundation, 1999; Simopoulos, 1999a; American Heart Association, 2001). Also, epidemiological evidence began to associate diets containing omega-3 fatty acids with a reduction in the risk of CHD and with a decline in all causes of mortality (Bang, Dyerberg, and Sinclair, 1980; Kromhout, Bosschieter, and de Lezenne Coulander, 1985; Hennekens, Buring, and Mayrent, 1990; Pauletto et al., 1996; Lorgeril et al., 1996).

Since the 1950s numerous studies have reported on the low incidence of atherosclerosis (fat deposition in the artery walls) in the Inuit nation from Greenland and in others from Norway in spite of their high lipid intakes, mainly DHA and EPA (Nettleton, 1995). The Inuit consume lipids in quantities comparable to those of Western populations but have a significantly lower incidence of CHD than do Western societies. The difference is that the Inuit consume essentially only omega-3 fatty acids (present in fish, seal, and whale fat), while Westerners eat mainly omega-6 fatty acids (Adam, 1988; Liepa and Gorman, 1991; Simopoulos, 1999a).

Following the publication of these studies in the 1970s interest in determining the relationship between omega-3 fatty acids and CHD increased (Illingworth and Ullmann, 1990; Nettleton, 1995). Many epidemiological studies, including those of the Inuit of Greenland, fishing populations from Japan, and others from Holland and Sweden (Bang and Dyerberg, 1972; Bang, Dyerberg, and Hjorne, 1976; Illingworth and Ullmann, 1990), as well as a large number of controlled studies demonstrated that high quantities of omega-3 fatty acids in the diet are associated with changes in lipids and lipoprotein concentrations in the blood. In general, a decline in triglycerides and VLDL and a variable response in other lipoproteins have been found (Illingworth and Ullmann, 1990; Bruckner, 1992; British Nutrition Foundation, 1992; Ascherio and Willett, 1996).

The biological effects of omega-3 fatty acids were first determined through the inclusion of DHA and EPA in the diet, with the first controlled research that positively correlated EPA with the prevention of thrombosis and arteriosclerosis conducted by Dyerberg et al. (1978). Later, in vitro work showed that although EPA and DHA had positive effects on placatory aggregation, EPA provided a greater inhibitory action (Simopoulos, 1988). The potential effects of alpha-linolenic acid remained untested for a long time, and only recently was attention turned to this source (McLennan and Dallimore, 1994). A reason for this could be that the only readily available source of alpha-linolenic acid was flaxseed (Horrobin, 1988), which is primarily used by industry rather than in human nutrition due to the antinutritional and toxic factors it contains.

Research published from 1986 onward has shown that increased alpha-linolenic acid in the diet, combined with decreased SFAs, is associated with a decline in platelet aggregation (thrombosis risk reduction), triglyceride levels, and blood pressure (Berry and Hirsch, 1986; Hunter, 1988; Emken, Adlof, and Gulley, 1994; Turini et al., 1994; Schaefer et al., 1996; Djousse et al., 2003). In 1995 research funded by the Australian National Health and Medical Research Council showed that a higher content of alpha-linolenic acid in the diet increased the EPA content in human tissues in a predictable manner. A linear relationship was determined between the incorporation of alpha-linolenic acid of vegetable origin and EPA concentrations in plasma and cellular phospholipids (Mantzioris et al., 1995). Research published in 1997 by the American Society for Clinical Nutrition compared the effects of supplying alpha-linolenic acids of vegetable origin with those produced by DHA and EPA from marine sources on hemostatic factors in humans. Differences could not be proven to be statistically different (Freese and Mutanen, 1997).

The protective effects of omega-3 fatty acids over thrombosis and arteriosclerosis is of special interest for diabetics because they are at increased risk from CHD. Borkman et al. (1993) showed that hyperinsulinemia and insulin resistance are inversely associated with the amount of EPA and DHA fatty acids in muscle cell membrane phospholipids in patients with CHD and in normal volunteers. High dietary intake of linoleic acid leads to increased production of arachidonic acid and interferes with the desaturation and elongation of alpha-linolenic acid to EPA and DHA. This increases the risk of CHD for diabetic patients (Bjerve et al., 1988).

Also, a number of epidemiological and controlled studies support the theory that consumption of alpha-linolenic omega-3 fatty acids is associated with a reduced risk of CHD (Lorgeril et al., 1994; Simon et al., 1995; Ferretti and Flanagan, 1996; Loria and Padgett, 1997; Li et al., 1999; Hu et al., 1999; Guallar et al., 1999; von Sharky et al., 1999; GISSI, 1999; Mantzioris et al., 2000; Iso et al., 2001; Ridges et al., 2001; Djousse et al., 2003). Controlled research has determined the minimum and optimum requirements of alpha-linolenic acid for an adult to be 0.2–1.2 percent of total calories consumed (Bjerve et al., 1988).

Long-chain Omega-3 Fatty Acids—DHA and EPA. The main source of DHA and EPA is fish oil. Not all fish oils are good sources of these fatty acids, and large variations have been observed. Salmon, tuna, sardines, trout, and corvina are among the species that have higher levels of these omega-3 fatty acids (Nettleton, 1995; Andrade et al., 1995; Tornaritis et al., 1994).

The beneficial effects of long-chain PUFAs have received much attention. However, EPA and DHA are more readily oxidized and result in more toxic oxidation products being formed than do linoleic, alpha-linolenic, and arachidonic acids (Cho et al., 1987). Studies have shown that EPA and DHA are able to reduce the risk of CHD, but only if antioxidative protection is sufficient to minimize undesirable lipid peroxidation and the disruption of the antioxidant system of cell membranes (Song, Fujimoto, and Miyazawa, 2000).

The need to add antioxidants to oils containing DHA is not just to prevent oxidation before delivery as an omega-3 fatty acid source but also to maintain stability after being consumed. A significant reduction of the alpha-tocopherol content in plasma and the liver has been reported when DHA oil was eaten. Because of the high susceptibility of DHA to peroxidation, more tissue alpha-tocopherol in the diet is required to protect tissue lipids from oxidative damage (Song and Miyazawa, 2001). The higher stability of alpha-linolenic acid compared with EPA and DHA is very important for human health. There is a close relationship between peroxidation and cardiovascular diseases and with other diseases such as cancer, cataracts, immune system decline, and brain dysfunction.

One advantage of consuming alpha-linolenic acid from plant sources, compared to EPA and DHA from marine sources, is that insufficient antioxidant intake does not exist at higher intakes (Simopoulos, 1999a). That is, we can eat as much alpha-linolenic acid as we want and not experience any problem, but if we consume too much EPA and DHA we can have peroxidation problems. There is scientific evidence of a direct association between lipid peroxidation and the progression of human atherosclerosis (Nishi et al., 2002). As was recently demonstrated by Song, Fujimoto, and Miyazawa (2000), DHA, when used to decrease the risk of atherosclerosis, can be transformed into a promoter of this disease if an imbalance between it and the amount of antioxidants present exists.

Another concern with increasing EPA levels as a source of omega-3 fatty acids is the potential for adverse immunological effects resulting from excessive intakes. A moderate to high amount of EPA but not of alpha-linolenic acid can decrease natural killer (NK) cell activity in healthy subjects (Thies et al., 2001). NK cells play an important role in defense against virus infections and in immune surveillance against tumor cells (Lewis and McGee, 1992).

Although there are variations between the recommendations made by nutritionists regarding the relationship among different omega-3 acids in the diet, nutritionists agree that the alpha-linolenic content must be significantly higher than the DHA content and within the range that these fatty acids exist in human milk. Breast milk has a DHA to alpha-linolenic ratio of 1:2.2, 1:2.2, 1:3.3, 1:3.6, 1:4, and 1:8 in women from Germany, France, Nigeria, Japan, China, and Nepal, respectively (Jensen and Lammi-Keefe, 1998; Yonekubo et al., 1998; Vander Jagt et al., 2000; Glew et al., 2001). In the United States the DHA to alpha-linolenic ratio in breast milk of women from Maryland, Connecticut, and Oklahoma was 1:4.4, 1:2.1, and 1:5, respectively (Bitman et al., 1981, and Henderson et al., 1992, cited in Nettleton, 1995; Jensen et al., 2000).

Today many government and private organizations are recommending an increase in omega-3 fatty acid intake. Since 1990 in Canada omega-3 fatty acids have been designated as essential nutrients, with the government issuing dietary recommendations for omega-3 fatty acids. They are to comprise at least 0.5 percent of total energy consumption (0.56 gram per 1,000 calories). In the United Kingdom the Department of Health (1991) recommended omega-3 PUFA intake based on energy intake, with a minimum of 0.2 percent of energy to come from these sources. The British Nutrition Foundation (1999) established minimum and maximum values for individuals as well as average intakes as follows: 0.5 and 2.5 percent of energy as a minimum and maximum for alpha-linolenic acids and 2 percent of energy as the maximum from long-chain omega-3 PUFAs (EPA and DHA). In the United States an official recommendation has not been established for omega-3 fatty acid intake. However, on 3 October 2000 the Food and Drug Administration (FDA) approved part 101 of the *Code of Federal Regulations*, title 21 (21 CFR Part 101), which allows food supplement labeling to claim that a beneficial action of omega-3 fatty acids is decreased risk of CHD (Food and Drug Administration, 2000).

Alpha-linolenic Acid versus EPA and DHA. Humans of all ages, including preterms and very likely fetuses, convert alpha-linolenic acid to DHA (Brenna, 2002; Billeaud et al., 1997). This process has been observed in other species as well (Ayerza and Coates, 2000). The conversion efficiency within species and between species is not well documented (Simopoulos, 2002); hence, the most convenient way to provide omega-3 fatty acids to humans and animals is not clear. Early theories came from minimal scientific knowledge about the biochemistry and physiologic functions of omega-3 fatty acids in general and of alpha-linolenic acid in particular. It was generally accepted that alpha-linolenic acid was just a precursor of long-chain polyunsaturated fatty acids, because the first epidemiological studies were conducted in populations having high fish intakes (Lauritzen et al., 2001).

Recent results, however, are changing our concept of omega-3 sources. Evidence from vegetarians shows that they do not suffer from diets that contain no DHA (Kwok et al., 2000; Li et al., 1999). Williard et al. (2001) found that as quantities of dietary DHA increased, DHA synthesis was reduced but not suppressed, even when the DHA level increased to very high concentrations. This is consistent with data from Ezaki, Takahashi, and Shigematsu (1999), who found a serum increase in DHA after ten months of feeding alpha-linolenic acid to elderly volunteers (age 67–91) in Japan. The authors were surprised, since the regular intake of long-chain omega-3 fatty acids from fish was considerable in these volunteers. Williard et al. (2001) concluded that some DHA synthesis persists even when excess DHA is available. This suggests that DHA synthesis from alpha-linolenic acid is a constitutive process that is required to fulfill an essential function in the brain.

Recently, Fu and Sinclair (2000) conducted a controlled experiment with guinea pigs and found that alpha-linolenic acid may have a function in relation to fur, perhaps as a lipid secreted from sebaceous glands to protect it from damage by water, light, and other agents. They concluded that if there is a substantial excretion of this fatty acid via sebaceous glands in humans, it might account for why alpha-linolenic acid rarely accumulates in most tissues. Substantial quantities of alpha-linolenic acid in the skin suggest that these could be potentially important reservoirs of omega-3 in the body. Yli-Jama et al. (2001) determined that a significant correlation between the percentage of alpha-linolenic acid in adipose tissue and in serum free fatty acids exists, as does the relationship between intake and concentration in adipose tissue of humans.

Omega-6 Fatty Acids. Nearly eighty years have passed since omega-6 fatty acids were identified as being an essential nutrient for laboratory animals.

Later they were shown to be essential for humans as well (Bjerve et al., 1988). Omega-6 PUFAs are present in many vegetable oils used in food and nutritional formulas (Taraszewaski and Jensen, 1994). The main commercial oils that supply omega-6 PUFAs and the percentage they contain are peanut (34 percent), soybean (54 percent), cotton (54 percent), corn (61 percent), sunflower (69 percent), and safflower (78 percent). In the mid-1990s a new flax variety named solin in Canada and linola in Australia came on the market. It contains 72 percent linoleic acid and less than 5 percent alpha-linolenic acid (White, 1992; Lin, 1996; Bell, 1996).

Omega-6 PUFAs were of interest for many years because of their capacity to lower cholesterol levels when compared with SFAs (Liepa and Gorman, 1991). In general, it was observed that diets rich in omega-6 PUFAs decrease blood cholesterol levels (Hegsted et al., 1965; Keys, Anderson, and Grande, 1965). These studies predicted that omega-6 PUFAs would lower blood cholesterol at twice the rate that SFAs increase it. Unfortunately, recent studies have demonstrated that omega-6 PUFAs also reduce HDL levels (Grundy, Barrett-Connor, and Rudel, 1988; Bruckner, 1992). Today the major effort in omega-6 PUFA research is focused on determining their effects compared to those of omega-3 PUFAs, due to the excessively high omega-6 fatty acid content of Western diets (Liepa and Gorman, 1991; British Nutrition Foundation, 1999).

There is evidence that increased intake of omega-6 fatty acids, particularly when associated with an elevated omega-6 to omega-3 fatty acid ratio, rather than serum cholesterol is a major risk factor leading to CHD (Okuyama, 2001). The British Nutrition Foundation (1992) concluded that partial replacement of SFAs by omega-6 PUFAs in the diet can reduce the risk of CHD, but it did not conclude that they can decrease the risk of death by all causes. It recommends that healthy adults limit their consumption of omega-6 PUFAs to a maximum of 6 percent of daily total energy (British Nutrition Foundation, 1992). In the United States recent recommendations suggest maintaining omega-6 PUFAs at 7 percent of total dietetic energy (Taraszewaski and Jensen, 1994).

The Ratio of Dietary Omega-6 to Omega-3 Fatty Acids. In most Western countries levels of dietary omega-3 PUFAs are quite low compared to omega-6 levels (Lands, 1992). This is reflected in the fatty acid balance of the plasma and other tissues (Simopoulos, 2003). The report *1994–96 Con-*

tinuing Survey of Food Intakes by Individuals, published by the United States Department of Agriculture (1997), showed the average omega-6 to omega-3 relationship to be 10:1.

Eicosanoids are a group of compounds that have a wide range of regulatory actions in the body. They produce smooth muscle constriction and promote blood clotting, cause both constriction and dilation of blood vessels and hence affect blood pressure, and mediate inflammatory and immunological responses. Omega-3 and omega-6 PUFAs compete for the same enzymes required in the desaturation and elongation processes in eicosanoid production and for their incorporation into fat tissues. Two eicosanoids, the prostacyclins and the thromboxanes, have essentially opposite physiological effects. Prostacyclins are among the most powerful inhibitors at preventing small blood components called platelets to clump together and form blood clots. They also have the effect of relaxing the walls of the arteries and hence lowering blood pressure. Thromboxanes are produced by platelets. They increase the tendency for platelets to aggregate and cause contraction of arterial walls, hence promoting an increase in blood pressure. The balance between these two opposite effects is important in maintaining normal blood vessel function.

Increased omega-6 fatty acids in the diet increase the quantity of eicosanoid metabolic products formed, specifically prostaglandins, thromboxanes, leukotrienes, hydroxy fatty acids, and lipoxins. Fewer of these are formed if omega-3 fatty acids, especially EPA, are increased in the diet. Thus, a diet rich in omega-3 fatty acids shifts the physiologic state to one that is antithrombotic and antiaggregatory. For this reason it is important to maintain a good relationship between omega-6 and omega-3 fatty acids in the diet. Based on present consumption levels of PUFAs, omega-6 fatty acid consumption must be reduced if an adequate relationship between these two groups of fatty acids is to be obtained and optimal human health achieved (British Nutrition Foundation, 1999; Simopoulos, Leaf, and Salem, 2000). Evidence also shows that an increased intake of omega-6 fatty acids when associated with an elevated omega-6 to omega-3 fatty acid ratio rather than with serum cholesterol is a major risk factor leading to CHD (Okuyama, 2001).

A workshop entitled "Essentiality of and Recommended Dietary Intakes for Omega-6 and Omega-3 Fatty Acids" was held at the Cloisters, the National Institute of Health (NIH), in Bethesda, Maryland, in 1999.

TABLE 2.5. Adequate intakes for adults on a 2,000-calorie diet

Fatty acid	g/day	% energy
Linoleic	4.44	2
(Upper limit)	6.67	3
Alpha-linolenic	2.22	1
DHA + EPA	0.65	0.3
DHA to be at least	0.22	0.1
EPA to be at least	0.22	0.1
Trans (upper limit)	2	1
Saturated (upper limit)	—	<8
MUFA	—	—

Source: Simopoulos, Leaf, and Salem, 2000.

The workshop participants stressed the need to reduce omega-6 fatty acid consumption and increase omega-3 fatty acid consumption in adult and newborn diets in order to promote optimal brain and cardiovascular health and function (Simopoulos, Leaf, and Salem, 2000). Tables 2.5 and 2.6 show the group's recommendations for adequate intakes of dietary fatty acids for adults and infants, respectively.

Evidence showing the beneficial effects of increased omega-3 fatty acid consumption has led to modifications in the nutritional policies of governments and other agencies. The United Nations, through both the Food and Agriculture Organization and the World Health Organization, has recommended adjusting the ratio of linoleic acid to alpha-linolenic acid consumption down from 10:1 to 5:1 (Food and Agriculture Organization, 1994; World Health Organization, 2003). The British Nutrition Foundation has recommended increasing omega-3 fatty acids in general and alpha-linolenic acids in particular to provide a ratio of 1:5 with linoleic acid (British Nutrition Foundation, 1999). The Canadian government, through its Department of Health and Welfare, has recommended decreasing the intake of omega-6 PUFAs to bring omega-6 to omega-3 consumption into equal proportions (Canada [Department of] Health and Welfare, 1990).

Trans-fatty Acids

The greatest amount of trans-fatty acids in the diet comes from processed vegetable oils. These oils initially have all double bonds in the cis position, but when they are heated with metal catalyzers to produce margarine and

TABLE 2.6. Adequate intakes for infants on a formula diet

Fatty acid	% fatty acid
Linoleic	10
Alpha-linolenic	1.5
Arachidonic	0.5
DHA	0.35
EPA (upper limit)	<0.10

Source: Simopoulos, Leaf, and Salem, 2000.

vegetable butters in a process called hydrogenation, the position changes (Ascherio and Willett, 1996). As this transformation comes about in commercial processes these trans-fatty acids are not considered natural and differ from the trans isomers of milk and meat, which are modified through biohydrogenation in the ruminant's body (Craig-Schmidt, 1992).

Partial hydrogenation is used by industry to obtain more solid, stable products from oils that have medium to high contents of unsaturated fatty acids such as soybean, sunflower, safflower, corn, and canola, making them physically similar to highly saturated fatty acids (Nettleton, 1995; Food and Agriculture Organization, 1994). The extent of hydrogenation depends on the unsaturated fatty acid content of the oil and the desired stability and physical properties of the final product, since hydrogenation increases stability and melting point (Nettleton, 1995; Food and Agriculture Organization, 1994; Emken, 1995). Hydrogenated vegetable oils used for cooking, baking, and frying are the main source of trans-fatty acids in a number of countries, including the United States and the United Kingdom (Cantwell, 2000).

Following the discovery of the hydrogenation process at the beginning of the last century, production and consumption of trans-fatty acids steadily increased up to the 1960s, with margarine replacing butter and pork fat in U.S. diets. Since 1960 trans-fatty acid consumption has decreased slightly, due to greater use of soft margarines, which generally have fewer trans isomers than bar or hard margarines (Ascherio and Willett, 1996; Aro et al., 1998). A similar sequence of events took place in other countries such as India and Pakistan, where partially hydrogenated oils containing 60 percent or more trans isomers became widely used, replacing the traditional ghee, which is of animal origin (Ascherio and Willett, 1996).

In countries with a large fishing industry marine oils are an important source of trans-fatty acids, because fish oil requires hydrogenation to improve stability. Partially hydrogenated fish oils are an important source of trans isomers in countries like Holland, Norway, Great Britain, Chile, Peru, and South Africa (Molketin and Precht, 1995; Innis and King, 1999). Hydrogenated or partially hydrogenated fish oil not only is a source of trans-fatty acids but also is a poor source of long-chain omega-3 fatty acids, since hydrogenation reduces EPA and DHA contents to less than 2 percent of total fat (Valenzuela and Uauy, 1999).

There is consistent evidence that supports the adverse effects on human health of trans-fatty acids, including increased risk of CHD (Ascherio and Willett, 1996; Cantwell, 2000). A number of studies have demonstrated that trans isomers increase blood cholesterol levels but somewhat less so than saturated fatty acids (Nettleton, 1995; Mensink and Katan, 1990; Judd et al., 1994; Lichtenstein, 1999). Recent research implies that trans-fatty acids may be worse than was previously thought because they not only increase LDL levels but also decrease HDL levels (Mensink and Katan, 1990; Judd et al., 1994). Another problem is that trans-fatty acids have an adverse effect on the metabolism of PUFAs under low intakes of PUFAs. Unlike saturated fatty acids, they compete for desaturation and elongation enzymes, interfering with omega-3 and omega-6 metabolism and inducing significant deficiencies of these essential fatty acids (Holman et al., 1994).

Since 1994 the United Nations has recommended excluding trans isomers from unsaturated fatty acids in human diets (Food and Agriculture Organization, 1994). The British Nutrition Foundation (1992) recommended that these isomers not exceed 2 percent of total energy consumption. The *Report of the Dietary Guidelines Advisory Committee on the Dietary Guidelines for Americans, 2000* (United States Department of Agriculture, 2000) recommends that the government emphasize avoidance of food sources containing trans-fatty acids and that it provide clear advice about how and why to limit trans fat consumption.

The Mediterranean Diet and CHD

Simopoulos and Visioli (2000) reported major differences among dietary patterns and health of people living in the countries surrounding the Mediterranean. They demonstrated that there is not one Mediterranean diet but in fact many Mediterranean diets. This is not surprising, as sixteen countries have shores on the Mediterranean Sea. Their populations represent a large variation in cultures, ethnic origins, religions, and economic and social development, all of which influence habits and nutrition. Simopoulos and Visioli thus concluded that the term "Mediterranean diet" is a misnomer.

"Mediterranean diet" has been used generically to refer to a diet characterized by an abundance of fruits, vegetables, breads and cereals, potatoes, legumes, and nuts and seeds and minimal quantities of processed foods. Fresh fruits are typical desserts, sweet desserts made with sugar or honey are consumed only a few times a week, olive oil is the main fat source, milk products (mainly yogurt and cheese) are consumed in moderate quantities, fish and chicken are eaten in moderate to low quantities, four eggs or fewer are consumed each week, low quantities of red meats are eaten, and moderate to low quantities of wine are served with meals (Willet et al., 1995; Nestle, 1995c).

The low incidence of CHD detected in people consuming the so-called Mediterranean diet was noted after the end of the Second World War, when in 1948 the government of Greece, conscious of the need to improve the social, economic, and sanitary conditions of the country, invited the Rockefeller Foundation to conduct an epidemiological study on the island of Crete. The study, published in 1953, determined that the composition of the diet and the low incidence of CHD were related (Nestle, 1995a). The diet represents the traditional Greek diet before 1960 and resembles a Paleolithic diet in terms of the quantities of antioxidants, fiber, saturated fats, and monounsaturated fats and the ratio of omega-6 to omega-3 fatty acids consumed (Simopoulos, 2001). Early on, when the beneficial effects of the Mediterranean diet were being attributed to oleic acid, what was not taken into account was three other fatty acids in the diet, all of which have been demonstrated to have a close relationship with CHD. These are saturated, polyunsaturated, and trans polyunsaturated fatty acids.

Certainly, components generally responsible for decreasing blood cholesterol were present in small quantities in the Mediterranean diet (James, 1995). Omega-3 polyunsaturated acids were not reported as being constituents of the Mediterranean diet, since they were consumed in small quantities and came from sources such as nuts and purslane (Renaud et al., 1995). Omega-3 fatty acids are known depressors of VLDL levels, triglycerides, and blood cholesterol (Howard et al., 1995). What was not considered was that this diet had minimal quantities of trans-fatty acids (James, 1995). These have recently been identified as being responsible for increasing blood cholesterol (Ascherio and Willett, 1996).

Greek society of the 1960s, the time when the Mediterranean diet was defined, had very different life habits from today. One of the most important differences is physical activity. In the 1960s most Greeks were physically very active, principally because of the kind of work they did. Other lifestyle differences include sharing long meals with friends and family, thereby allowing time to relax and rest from daily stress, and taking daily naps, which provide an extra opportunity to relax and rest (Willet et al., 1995; Renaud et al., 1995). Physical exercise and lack of stress have been identified as important factors in reducing the risk of CHD.

The low incidence of CHD in Crete compared with Western countries caused many to conclude that the difference was due to diet. Large publicity campaigns expounded on the healthy benefits of daily consumption of this or that product that was a "fundamental part of the Mediterranean diet," with the result being fewer heart attacks. In 1993 Harvard University organized an international conference on the Mediterranean diet. This event brought together seventy scientists and experts in nutrition, diet, and health who analyzed and discussed a wide range of research topics related to the description, definition, history, perceptive quality, and effects on health of the Mediterranean diet as well as the political implications regarding patterns attributed to it. The *American Journal of Clinical Nutrition* published the work in 1995, and it represented virtually all available information on the nutrition and health of the Mediterranean region at that time.

Although the report gave solid support to the health benefits of eating a vegetable-based diet, it also demonstrated that many aspects of diet-health relationships were tied to other factors such as type of agriculture, combination of foods eaten, and environmental factors (Nestle, 1995a; James, 1995; Ferro-Luzzi and Branca, 1995; Helsing, 1995; Katan, Zock, and Mensink, 1995). An example is mechanization. In Crete mechanization has essentially eliminated the need to do heavy physical tasks. This in turn has increased obesity, which is closely related to CHD (Katan, Zock, and Mensink, 1995).

Early observations suggested that legumes and olive oil were responsible for the low incidence of CHD in Crete. Later work demonstrated that the Mediterranean diet also contains significant quantities of alpha-linolenic omega-3 fatty acid. This has been shown to markedly reduce mortality due to CHD (Lorgeril et al., 1994; Djousse et al., 2003). Thus the Mediterranean diet is considered beneficial in lowering the risk of CHD, but this comes about not only because of reduced saturated fat and cholesterol levels and increased monounsaturated fats but also because of the presence of omega-3 fatty acids (Sacks, 1998; Lorgeril et al., 1994, 1996). New scientific evidence clearly shows that the diet of Crete included not only omega-3 fatty acids but also a number of other beneficial components such as high amounts of fiber, antioxidants, and vitamins E and C as well as a balanced ratio of omega-6 to omega-3 fatty acids, giving the diet its healthy properties (Simopoulos, 2001).

THREE

A Hidden Food of the Americas

Chia was one of the most important crops of the Aztecs at the time of the Spanish conquest. This chapter attempts to explain why, following the collapse of the Aztec Empire, chia lost its importance and essentially disappeared from Mexican culture. The information that was gathered to do this came from various historical records, with the documentation divided into five categories: codices (*códices*), or manuscripts written before Columbus; sixteenth-century scrolls written in a native language but using Latin characters; sixteenth-century scrolls written in Spanish and Latin; seventeenth-century texts written in Spanish and Italian; and modern historical and archaeological reports. The first two categories are native sources; the third contains information obtained by individuals who had direct contact with natives during the first few years following the conquest; the fourth is considered historical research and is based on previously written documents that are no longer available; the last is a combination of information obtained by studying documents in the four other categories and then combining this with archaeological investigations.

When it was not possible to access the original documents, reproductions recognized as being authentic were consulted. Only the historical reports of authors who are known to be of unquestionable reliability were used. When the original material was in Spanish or Italian, this was translated by us with the help of friends, except where noted otherwise. Their help is acknowledged.

Mesoamerica and the Origin of the Nahua People

The Spanish word "Mesoamerica" is used by archaeologists and historians to describe the region where sophisticated pre-Columbian civilizations, including the Archaic, Olmec, Teotihuacán, Toltec, Maya, Mixtec, Zapotec, and Aztec, were situated. All of these peoples had cultural similarities. Mesoamerica extended from 100 miles north of Mexico City (called Tenochtitlán City in Aztec times) to the northern part of what today is Costa Rica and included parts of Belize, El Salvador, Guatemala, Honduras, and Nicaragua (León Portilla, 1971; MacLaren and Sugiura, 1991; García Cook, 1992). The region was defined not only by geographic limits, with its center being the Central Valley of Mexico, but also by its ethnic composition and cultural practices. Many of these similarities were related to the use and cultivation of various plants, with Paul Kirchhoff listing some: "a certain type of digging-stick (coa); the construction of gardens by reclaiming land from lakes (chinampas); the cultivation of lime-leaved sage (chia) and its use for a beverage and for oil to give luster to paints; the cultivation of the century plant (maguey) for its juice (aguamiel), fiber for clothing and paper, and maguey beer (pulque); the cultivation of cacao; the grinding of corn softened with ashes or lime" (1943:92).

The Teotihuacán civilization (100 B.C.–A.D. 850) planned, built, and administered a human wonder, that is, the city that carried its name. Its cultural and economic influence was based on natural resources and commerce, combined with the production and distribution of agricultural goods. Advanced agricultural technology, including massive irrigation and terracing projects, made intensive cultivation possible. Because of this it was able to feed the 200,000 inhabitants living in the urban center that served as the hub of this civilization (MacLaren and Sugiura, 1991; Whitmore and Turner, 1992).

After the collapse of Teotihuacán, the Toltecs made their appearance on the Mesoamerican stage. The Toltec Empire grew quickly, extending its control and economic influence over most of northern Mesoamerica between 700 B.C. and A.D. 1165. Militarism and control of the irrigation in the Valley of Tula have been suggested as the key components that contributed to the empire's growth, allowing it to control most of Central Mexico (MacLaren and Sugiura, 1991; Matos Moctezuma, 1994).

The Aztecs, who were also known as Mexicas, came to the valley from a place called Aztlán to the north. It is from this name that the people became known as Aztecs. Although the exact location of Aztlán has not been precisely identified, it is thought to have been located where the Mexican states of Jalisco, Guanajuato, and Michoacán are today. The Aztec civilization was at its maximum splendor between 1168 and 1521 but then was destroyed by the Spanish conquerors, led by Hernán Cortés, with the support of rebellious Indian allies (Cortés, 1522; Hernández, 1575; Solís, 1770; Matos Moctezuma, 1994).

The Aztecs spoke Nahuatl (Lorenzana, 1770); however, Nahuatl was the language of many other groups as well. It was the common language of the entire Valley of Mexico, which was comprised of many city-states, including the fabled cities of Toltec, Tula, and probably Teotihuacán. Today more than a million people distributed over the central part of Mexico speak Nahuatl and are commonly called Nahuas. These people, as their ancestors did, call themselves Mexicas.

When Christopher Columbus landed in America the Aztec civilization controlled a large portion of Mesoamerica and had a population of more than 11 million. Three million were living in the Valley of Mexico (McCaa, 1995). In his many trips to conquer the interior of the region and while looking for the capital of the Aztec Empire, Cortés (1522) described the numerous crowded towns and cities through which he passed: Amaqueruca (20,000 inhabitants), Iztapalpa (12,000–15,000 inhabitants), and Texcoco (30,000 inhabitants), to name a few. In a letter written to Charles I of Spain and Germany Cortés gave his impression of the enormous population: "There is such a large number of people living in these places that there is not an inch that has not been ploughed, and still, many people are starving because of a shortage of bread. The poor are begging among the rich in the streets, homes, and markets like poor people do in Spain and other places where intelligent people can be found" (1522:79).

During the thirteenth century the Aztecs established the capital city of Tenochtitlán, located where Mexico City is today. It had 200,000 inhabitants, twice the population of the contemporary cities of London and Rome. The market of Tlatelolco, along with the one in Tenochtitlán, at tracted a thousand people a day (Díaz del Castillo, 1568; Hernández, 1575; Matos Moctezuma, 1994). Cortés described the main Tenochtitlán market: "There is another huge square as big as the city of Salamanca. It is surrounded by arcades where about sixty thousand souls trade every day. All kinds of goods can be found there, from maintenance goods to provisions" (1522:80). Cortés was impressed not only by the size of the Temixtitlán market, as he called the Aztec capital, but also by the tremendous variety of products found there: "In these markets all goods found on Earth are sold. Apart from the ones I have already mentioned there is such an immense variety of goods that I ran short of words to describe them, and I cannot possibly remember what they are and what they are called" (1522:81).

Tenochtitlán covered an area of some 10 square miles, several times larger than sixteenth-century London, and was built on an island in the center of Lake Texcoco. It was connected to the mainland by a series of broad causeways, supplied with fresh water by means of a huge aqueduct, and surrounded by floating agricultural plots called *chinampas*. The high towers and painted buildings rising from the water sparkled in the sunlight and made a great impression on Cortés and his companions, who asked themselves if they were dreaming (Díaz del Castillo, 1568; Sahagún, 1579). In 1522 Cortés set its size as being equal to the Spanish cities of Seville and Cordova combined and said that its prominent buildings were more grandiose than the castle of Burgos. Thus, Tenochtitlán, the capital city of the Aztec Empire, was one of the wonders of the ancient world.

Francisco Hernández, a doctor, in his manuscript entitled *Antigüedades de la Nueva España* (*Antiquities of New Spain*), which was written in Latin and prepared at the request of Philip II of Spain in 1575, described the grandiosity of the city of Texcoco, which contained 100,000 inhabitants. In this historic work, which today is housed in the Biblioteca de la Real Academia de la Historia in Madrid, Hernández wrote: "The houses are placed in every direction and separated one from the other, just as in every other city in New Spain. Like in most towns, the houses are surrounded by parcels of land in which corn, amaranth, chia, chile, pumpkins, beans, and the like are cultivated. In this way you will not see cities but the Orchards of Hesperides and charming fields that spread out over the horizon, especially if the suburbs are added to it" (1575:130).

Sixteenth-century scrolls discovered during the second half of the twentieth century, combined with recent archaeological discoveries, throw new light on the Aztec civilization. There are no doubts that the Nahua nations possessed a wonderful form of architecture, exhibited pure forms of art, sculpture, and painting, and had an exact knowledge of time expressed in two calendars. In addition, a complex religion, fair and at the same time strict rights, well-developed commerce, a powerful and disciplined army, an elaborate educational system, and a deep knowledge of botany applied for food and health purposes existed. This was one of the great civilizations of the world (Soustelle, 1955; León Portilla, 1966; MacLaren and Sugiura, 1991).

Given the advanced state of the Nahua world in the sixteenth century, we can begin to understand the confusion and at the same time the admiration that the Aztec civilization inspired in the comparatively crude soldiers who accompanied Cortés. Those feelings were documented in sixteenth-century scrolls handwritten by soldiers, accompanying religious leaders, and others who collected testimonials during the European advance (Cortés, 1522; Las Casas, 1552; Cervantes de Salazar, 1554; Díaz del Castillo, 1568; Durán, 1570; Hernández, 1575; Sahagún, 1579; Torquemada, 1615; Solís, 1770; Clavijero, 1780).

The Origin of Agriculture and Its Importance for Mesoamerican Cultures

Mesoamerica is considered one of the main origins and a center of domestication of plant species (Vavilov, 1931; Bye, 1993). Here agriculture was adopted later than in the Old World, perhaps as much as one thousand years later. There is evidence of agriculture existing in the Valley of Tehuacán, some 15 miles south of Mexico City, by 9000 B.C. Around 3400 B.C. corn, chia, amaranth, pumpkin, beans, chile, avocado, *zapote* (the common name of the plant *Achras zapota* L.), and several types of squash were brought into cultivation (Schery, 1972; Solbrig and Solbrig, 1990; Harlan, 1992; Rodríguez Vallejo, 1992).

The process of plant domestication is closely connected with the abandonment of a nomadic lifestyle and the adoption of a sedentary lifestyle. The existence of huge, sophisticated urban centers (Teotihuacán, Tula, Tenochtitlán, Tepeapac, Texcoco, and Tlatelolco in central Mexico; Palenque in southern Mexico; Copan in Honduras; and Tikal in Guatemala), which in many cases surpassed 250,000 inhabitants, would not have been possible without advanced agrarian development. This included planting a diverse range of species; cropping, harvesting, and storage systems; and a wide range of uses for the crops (León Portilla, 1966; Cuevas Sánchez, 1992; García Cook, 1992). Agriculture played a significant role in pre-Columbian American societies. It stabilized these highly developed cultures and influenced every facet of life in ancient Mesoamerica, from political and economic policies to the many gods worshiped (MacLaren and Sugiura, 1991; Estrada Lugo, 1992; García Cook, 1992; Matos Moctezuma, 1994).

The Aztecs made significant advances in agriculture. An example is their very unique system for growing amaranth, beans, chia, and corn in Lake Texcoco on man-made islands called hanging gardens, or *chinampas*. Using what they learned from their predecessors, the Toltecs, the Aztecs were able to turn the marshy ground into firm soil. To do this they wove bark from trees into large mats, attached them to stakes in the lake, and covered the mats with soil. At the edges of the plots a type of willow, *ahuexotl*, was planted; the roots became interwoven and prevented erosion of the plots.

According to some reports (Schilling, 1993; Tylor, 1993; Matos Moctezuma, 1994), this cropping system was introduced in Teotihuacán times. However, according to an Aztec document written in the hieroglyphic Nahua system that was interpreted by older natives and translated into Spanish by Fray Juan de Torquemada in 1615, the creation of this fantastic technology is attributed to the Aztecs themselves. Torquemada not only described the chinampas but also mentioned chia:

"On behalf of the king of Azcaputzalco, I command you to double the tribute and to produce a sown field at the same level of the water that would move like a raft and to grow the seeds that were used as sustenance, which are corn, chile, beans, pumpkins, chia, and some amaranths called Huauhtli." When the Mexicans learned about this they started to cry, and they were soon overcome by deep sadness. Breaking this new law meant their deaths. With this feeling they returned home, and they visited their god Huitzilopuhtli, whom they always turned to whenever they needed help, and presented him this new and tough imposition. He comforted them and told one of their priests: "Tell the Mexicans not to worry and to accept the tribute. I will help them. Tell my son, Acampichitli, to work hard and to take the Savins and the Willows where they are ordered to, to build the rafts on the water and to grow all the vegetables and seeds they are asked to on them, because I will make things easy for you." In this way they easily found the savins and the willows, they took them to Azaput-zalco, they planted them where Rei Tecocmoc had ordered them to be. They could easily find all the seeds and grow them properly. When the crops were ready, they were taken in these rafts just over the water to where the king was, as he had planned. When the king Tecocmoc saw this incredible plantation, he was astonished and told his court: "This is above humans' ability, my brothers. When I gave this commandment I never thought you would be able to put up with it. Bring all the Mexicans to me because I want to tell them that they have been favored by their god, and for that reason they shall be considered to be above all nations."

In addition to using chinampas for agricultural production the Aztecs also farmed the mountains surrounding the lake, as they were covered by agricultural terraces. These were irrigated with fresh water brought in by a sophisticated system of aqueducts and canals (MacLaren and Sugiura, 1991; Whitmore and Turner, 1992; Rojas Rabiela, 1993a).

The climate of the Central Valley of Mexico is semiarid, having a single rainy period in the summer. In addition to being concentrated over a short period of time, total rainfall varies significantly between years, with very dry seasons followed by others having significant rainfall. Under these climatic conditions the chinampas, combined with the irrigated terraces, allowed the Aztecs to make multiple harvests each year. This is quite different from a dry farming system, which allows only one harvest per year. These sophisticated agricultural systems allowed the Aztecs not only to overcome poor rain-fall distribution but also to produce surplus quantities of food that stored well and provided reserves for several seasons. This surplus was especially important for the poor, the old people, and the children, as described by Fray Diego Durán in 1570: "Given this order and commandment, twenty canoes carrying bread, ten carrying atole made from toasted corn flour and chia mixed, entered the city of Mexico. The king placed managers and dis-tributors, who brought the poor people from all neighborhoods together (children, adults, old people). They distributed the bread among them, con-sidering their different needs. The children were given a big bowl of atole" (1570:242).

Nahua texts translated into Spanish by Torquemada in 1615 describe the effects that rainy years, referred to as *toxiuhmolpia* in the Aztec calendar, had on Aztec agriculture: "That was a prosperous year. The abundant rainfall that year enabled them to grow corn, hauauhli, chian [chia], beans, and lots of other vegetables. Every peasant was totally satisfied. This is what tales and paintings from those times tell us."

The sudden collapses of the Teotihuacán civilization in the Central Valley of Mexico and the Mayan civilization in Central America at about the same time have not been satisfactorily explained. There are many hypotheses. One is that a natural catastrophe that lasted long enough to exhaust food reserves took place. Other theories include a revolt of the lower classes, disease, earthquakes, and economic factors. A long dry period would affect Teotihuacán culture by decreasing the availability of irrigation water. It would also affect the dryland farms of the Mayan milpa agricultural system by preventing the production of basic crops (Cancian, 1971; León Portilla, 1971; Benson, 1977; MacLaren and Sugiura, 1991).

There is evidence of extended dry periods and the resulting catastrophic effects on pre-Columbian civilizations. One occurred during the time when the Teotihuacán civilization was at its peak. Pollen data suggest that during the growth period of Teotihuacán culture conditions were favorable for agriculture but that dry conditions existed during the period in which this culture disappeared (McClung de Tapia, 1997). Another dry period occurred at the beginning of the fifteenth century and lasted four years. This affected agricultural production so significantly that thousands of people died. From 1453 to 1456, during the rule of Montezuma I, a dry period dramatically affected the Aztec economy (Cortés, 1522; Matos Moctezuma, 1989). Durán, through oral and written information obtained from the Aztecs, described this dry period in 1570: "1454 was considered the year *Cetochtli*, which means one rabbit, according to the Indians' counting system. The following two years the lack of water in those lands was such that the clouds seemed to be shut, and almost—as in Elías's time—it didn't rain, neither a little nor a lot, and the sky didn't show a will to provide them with water" (1570:241).

In Mesoamerica the occurrence of dry periods is a phenomenon that is repeated even today, such as from 2000 to 2001 in Honduras, El Salvador, Guatemala, and Nicaragua. During this time basic crops could not be harvested, government stocks were depleted, and it was necessary to import huge quantities of food. The severity of this situation was increased because another catastrophe, Hurricane Mitch, had struck in 1998. This hurricane not only damaged practically all crops but, worse yet, destroyed the infrastructure needed to maintain stable agricultural production. Reconstruction was not fast enough to bring the agricultural sector back to prehurricane production levels and rebuild the reserves prior to the second crisis, the drought. In August 2001 the Guatemalan government declared a national disaster due to a lack of food. Comparing the technological capabilities of 900 and 2001 and considering that the current population of Guatemala is just 25 percent larger than the one that occupied the eastern part of the country in 900, we can see why Tikal and other urban centers of the ancient Mayan civilization might have been in serious trouble. The only solution in 2001 was international help, with food from other regions of the world being sent to avoid countless deaths. Such an alternative was not available for these people's ancestors.

Today when famines occur farmers abandon their land and go to the cities. This occurred in Honduras during the 1980s. In pre-Columbian times just the opposite took place; when city food stocks declined the only alternative was to go to the forest in the hope of finding wild animals or plants that could be eaten. Durán described such an exodus when referring to the drought that occurred in the Central Valley of Mexico between 1454 and 1457, as related to him by Aztec wise men: "Eating unhealthy food, people started to grow ill. Others passed out and became unhealthy due to starvation. People started to leave the cities, their houses, and even their wives and children, looking for fertile lands and the cure to this terrible disease" (1579:241). Durán described what happened after Montezuma I informed his people that the food reserves were gone: "Bitterly crying, people left the cities and went to other places where they felt they had found some relief . . . a place that became their new home, a place where they nowadays still remain" (1579:243, 244).

Even with the extraordinary growing abilities that the Aztecs possessed in the fifteenth century, they were unable to produce sufficient reserves to carry on if more than three years' worth of crops were lost (Solís, 1770). Durán described in 1570 what the Aztecs said took place when such shortages occurred:

> After a year during which the king had given food to his people, there was such a shortage of food that the king could no longer support them the following year. He was told by his butlers that his granaries were running short of food, so he called every man and woman, old or young, and offered them a last banquet with the corn and the other seeds that were left in the city. Once they had

finished eating, he sent every man to be dressed in serape and *bragueros* [belt] and every woman in shirts and skirts. When this was over he delivered a comforting but exhortative talk. The people were really touched by his speech and started whimpering and crying. In his speech he said: "Dear sons and brothers, in these hard times, I appeal to your patience and suffering, for we didn't fight against our enemies in the fields. Had we fought against them, we would have risked our lives to defend ourselves, and we would have died complying with our duties. The one who is declaring war on us is the Lord of the servants, the night and the day. Who could defeat him? It is his will that there is no rain, that the land is heated, and that plants are burned, . . . something never seen or heard of before." (1570:242–43)

Besides suffering through adverse climatic conditions and having to farm the steep topography of the land, Mesoamerican farmers faced other equally limiting factors such as poor soils that greatly reduced yields. To overcome these limitations ancient Americans developed a series of very effective agricultural practices that today would be called conservation farming.

On the lowlands of the Yucatán peninsula the agricultural system that is still used today by descendants of the Maya is called milpa farming. This term is derived from the Nahua word for cornfield. Native trees are cleared and burned during the dry season, and the ashes are used as fertilizer. The crop is sown when the rainy season starts. Depending on soil fertility, the field is cropped for one to three years. The field is then abandoned, the farmers move to another area, and the process is repeated. Helped by heavy rainfall and high temperatures, the native vegetation soon covers the abandoned field.

Mayan and Nahua farmers did not plow the soil to sow their crops; rather, they used a digging stick for planting. They were not inverting the soil but only making holes for the seeds. Although some Mayan descendants are now using digging sticks with metal points, following the conquest most replaced the digging stick with plows (Cancian, 1971; Benson, 1977). Thus, a practice that had allowed cultivation to take place without inverting the soil was replaced by plows, which invert and mix the soil horizons. Five hundred years later the loss in soil fertility and the resulting decrease in crop yield show us why pre-Columbian growers used a zero-till system. By turning over the soil and not rotating agricultural crops with periods of permanent vegetation, production cannot be sustained.

Often Nahua and Mayan growers planted two crops in the same field at the same time. This practice, unknown in the Old World, favored better use of available soil nutrients. When corn and beans are grown together nitrogen is captured from the atmosphere by the beans and fixed in the soil by root nodules, thus making it available for use by both crops.

Based on efficient agricultural systems, ancient Americans developed advanced societies that at the beginning of the sixteenth century supported a Mesoamerican population of more than 11 million (McCaa, 1995). Today, Mesoamerica has almost the same number of people, 12.5 million, living in hunger (Food and Agriculture Organization, 2001). Most are farmers and descendants of the Nahua and Mayan nations who created the early sophisticated agricultural systems.

The Codices, Other Early Writings, and Chia

According to the dictionary of the Real Academia de la Lengua Española (Royal Academy of the Spanish Language), a codex (*códice*) is a book of historic or literary importance handwritten before the invention of the printing press. Most archaeologists and historians of Mesoamerica, however, refer to a codex as a book written by pre-Columbian cultures, with some having been reprinted by the conquerors at a later date.

The Aztecs developed all of the tools necessary to record their history. They had an elaborate writing system based on hieroglyphics and produced paper of an excellent quality called *amaquahuitl* (paper tree). They made the paper by peeling bark from different ficus trees (*Ficus petrolaris, F. cotinifolia, F. involuta,* and *F. padifolia*) and then hammering it into thin sheets with a mallet (Bonfil Batalla, 1987); they also made a paper called *metl* in Nahuatl or *pita* in Spanish using leaves from plants like maguey (*Agave* spp.) or palm (Lorenzana, 1770).

Unfortunately, very few pre-Columbian codices have survived. Among the exceptions are the *Matrícula de tributos* and the Codex Borbonicus. The first is in the Museo Nacional de Mexico; the second is held by the Bibliothèque nationale de Paris. The origin of the Codex Borbonicus is in dispute by historians.

The cultural differences that existed between ancient Americans and the Spanish conquerors led to an irreparable loss for humanity, that is, the knowledge developed over centuries by pre-Columbian nations. This loss took place through the destruction of the codices and by imposing one culture onto another. An example is that of Fray Francisco Diego de Landa, a Yucatán bishop. His act of faith in Mani in 1562 led to the destruction of five thousand idols and the burning of twenty-seven Mayan codices (Armando and Fantoni, 1997). It was not only the Spanish priests who destroyed Mesoamerican codices in an attempt to erase "heretical" customs but also Itzcoatl, the fourth Aztec king. In the fifteenth century Itzcoatl destroyed a great number of codices in an attempt to rewrite Aztec history and establish the Aztecs as the rightful heirs of the Toltec legacy, in admiration of their ancestors' accomplishments in the Valley of Mexico (MacLaren and Sugiura, 1991).

The books that the Spanish called codices were written shortly after the conquest. During the sixteenth century a number of these as well as dictionaries and histories of the Indians were produced by Catholic priests. These writings were compiled to help them understand the Indians and to ease their conversion to Catholicism (Sahagún, 1579; León Portilla, 1971; Matos Moctezuma, 1994).

One work that reveals Aztec customs is the Codex Mendoza, also known as the Codex Mendocino. It is a complex document containing historic, economic, and ethnographic information that was produced in Mexico City between 1541 and 1542, shortly after the conquest. It was written at the request of the first viceroy of New Spain, Antonio de Mendoza, by native scribes (*tlacuilos*) on European paper in straight Spanish (not in verse) and contains thirty-five colored illustrations. It is now in the Bodleian Library at Oxford University.

The Codex Mendoza is divided into three sections, with the second being a copy of the pre-Columbian codex known as the *Matrícula de tributos*. This lists the tributes such as corn, beans, chia, amaranth, and other goods that were paid annually to the Aztecs by conquered nations and includes the names of the places and the quantity paid by each (figure 3.1). As is documented in the Codex Mendoza, the city of Tenochtitlán received yearly tributes from conquered nations that amounted to thousands of tons of corn, beans, chia, and amaranth. In addition, the people of Tenochtitlán harvested an average of 3,335 tons of corn, chia, beans, and amaranth from the 9,000 hectares of chinampas surrounding the city (Parsons, 1993).

It is interesting to note that the most civilized people living in America

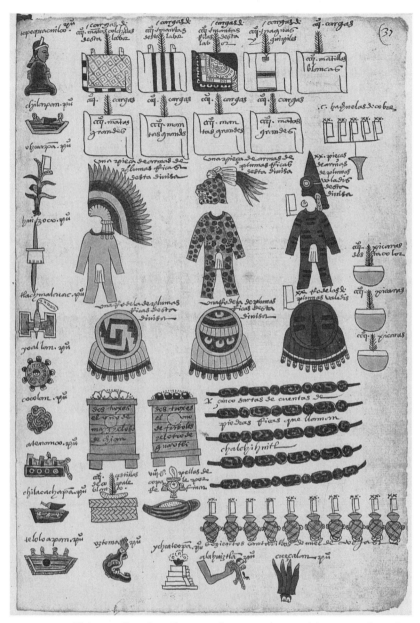

FIGURE 3.1. This page lists the tributes such as corn, beans, chia, amaranth, and other goods that were paid annually to the Aztecs by conquered nations and includes the names of places and the quantity paid by each. (From the Codex Mendoza, Courtesy of the Bodleian Library, Oxford University.)

when the Spanish arrived, the Aztecs in Mesoamerica and the Incas in South America, both cropped three of the four plants: corn, beans, and amaranth. The domestication processes that led these two civilizations to grow the same plants took place in parallel but were totally independent of one another (Parodi, 1935).

Molins Fábrega (1955) compiled a table showing the quantities and origin of the four main grain crops paid as tributes to Tenochtitlán as described in the Codex Mendoza. This table was published with the values expressed in *trojes*, a volume of measure used by the Nahua nations. Folio 21 of the Codex Mendoza, which was translated from Nahuatl into Spanish in the sixteenth century, talks about the conversion of trojes (or *troxes*) into *fanegas*: ". . . and four big wooden troxes [bins]. One was full of beans, the other was full of chian, the third was full of corn, and the fourth and last was full of guautli or amaranth seed. Each troxe could be filled with four and five thousands fanegas, which were paid as a tribute once a year."

In the sixteenth century different sizes of fanegas were used. Following extensive study, León Portilla (1971) selected the fanega from Castile, which is one of the smallest (55.5 liters), as being the most likely one used by the Aztecs. Using an average value of 4,500 fanegas per troje and Molins Fábrega's (1955) work, the tributes listed in the Codex Mendoza can be converted to liters. For this book the liters were then converted to weight using seed obtained from Valle de Lerma, Salta, Argentina. As amaranth is no longer produced in northwestern Argentina, the volume-to-weight calculation was made with seed purchased by the authors in the Lince market of Lima, Peru. From these data it was determined that a troje of maize, beans, chia, and amaranth weighed 234.8, 232.2, 204.8, and 108.5 tons, respectively. Table 3.1 was prepared using these values and those that Fábrega calculated from the Codex Mendoza.

The Codex Florentino, written between 1548 and 1579 by Fray Bernardino de Sahagún, was entitled *Historia general de las cosas de Nueva España* (General History of Things from New Spain). It is possible to discuss the Codex Florentino at great length, given the extraordinary quality of this work. Without doubt it has a fundamental place in the evaluation of pre-Columbian cultures (León Portilla, 1966, 1988; Gomez Pompa, 1993). The original twelve-volume set of books is held by the Biblioteca Medicea Laurenziana in Florence, Italy.

In the Codex Florentino Sahagún wrote in both Nahuatl and Spanish,

TABLE 3.1. Tributes from conquered nations delivered annually to Tenochtitlán

Province	Number of towns	Corn	Beans	Chia	Amaranth
		(t/year)			
Tepecuacuilco	14	234.8	232.2	204.8	180.5
Tlachco	10	234.8	—	204.8	—
Ocuilán	6	234.8	232.2	204.8	180.5
Tuluca	12	469.6	232.2	409.6	180.5
Malinalco	2	469.6	464.4	409.6	361
Quahuacán	13	234.8	232.2	204.8	180.5
Atotonilco de Pedraza	7	234.8	232.2	204.8	180.5
Quahuitlán	7	234.8	232.2	204.8	180.5
Xilotepec	7	234.8	232.2	204.8	180.5
Axocopán	10	234.8	232.2	204.8	180.5
Hueypuchtla	9	234.8	232.2	204.8	180.5
Atotonilco el Grande	6	234.8	232.2	204.8	180.5
Acolhuacán	26	234.8	232.2	204.8	180.5
Chalco	6	1,408.8	464.4	204.8	180.5
Quahuhnahuac	16	234.8	232.2	204.8	180.5
Huaxtepec	26	234.8	232.2	204.8	180.5
Tepeacac	22	469.6	464.4	—	—
Coyolapán	11	469.6	232.2	204.8	—
Petlacalco	23	234.8	232.2	204.8	180.5
Xocotitlán	1	234.8	232.2	204.8	180.5
Total/year		6,809	5,108	4,301	3,249

side by side on the same page. Neither the Spanish nor the Nahuatl is a translation from the other. In 1963 the Nahuatl side of the Codex Florentino was translated into English by Arthur J. O. Anderson and Charles Dibble. When we compared the original Spanish side and Anderson and Dibble's English translation from the Nahuatl, we found variations in content in many places. For this book most of the paragraphs taken from the Codex Florentino were translated from Spanish into English. However, when a paragraph from the Anderson and Dibble English translation seems to be more illustrative than the Spanish paragraph, the English translation was chosen.

Sahagún's objective in writing the Codex Florentino was to help teach the Catholic religion to the natives of the Valley of Mexico by better knowing their customs. Hence the Codex Florentino covers all of the basic subjects of native life and is considered the genuine encyclopedia of Nahuatl knowledge (León Portilla, 1966; Estrada Lugo, 1989, 1992; Matos Moctezuma, 1994). It describes the stage of development reached by the Aztecs

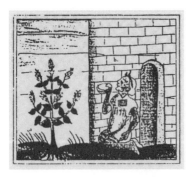 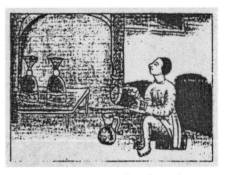

FIGURE 3.2. Drawing taken from the Codex Florentino (Sahagún, 1579) illustrating chia and one of its uses. (*Florentine Codex. General History of the Things of New Spain. Fray Bernardino de Sahagún.* Book 11. Translated and edited by Arthur J. O. Anderson and Charles E. Dibble. Santa Fe, New Mexico, and Salt Lake City: The School of American Research and The University of Utah Press, 1963. Reprinted courtesy of The University of Utah Press.)

FIGURE 3.3. Drawing taken from the Codex Florentino (Sahagún, 1579) illustrating the use of chia. (*Florentine Codex. General History of the Things of New Spain. Fray Bernardino de Sahagún.* Book 11. Translated and edited by Charles E. Dibble and Arthur J. O. Anderson. Santa Fe, New Mexico, and Salt Lake City: The School of American Research and The University of Utah Press, 1963. Reprinted courtesy of The University of Utah Press.)

and other Nahua nations in growing and using domesticated plants and covers in detail topics such as soil type and quality, methods of soil preparation for sowing, sowing methods, use of manure for fertilizer, harvesting, storage, agricultural tools and systems, crop uses, and marketing.

Many aspects of the production, commercialization, and use of chia by the Aztecs and their conquered nations are described in this monumental work. Sahagún refers to chia in six of the twelve books that compose the Codex Florentino: volume 2, calendars, festivities, sacrifices, and religious ceremonies; volume 5, the origin of the gods; volume 8, kings and the government; volume 9, merchants and crafts; volume 10, the human body, illness, and medicines; and volume 11, animals, plants, metals, and stones. A number of pictures illustrate chia and its uses; see figures 3.2 and 3.3 for two examples.

The characterization of the ecological regions and the crops grown by the Aztecs and the nations that were subject to them as reported in the Codex Florentino, combined with the Codex Mendoza's description of annual tributes, provides enormous information about the regions where chia was grown and the amounts produced at the time the Spaniards arrived in America.

The codex entitled *Historia de los indios de Nueva España e islas de la tierra firme* (History of the Natives of New Spain and the Islands of Terra Firma), written by Durán in the sixteenth century, is comprised of two volumes. They are now in the Biblioteca Nacional de Madrid. Durán arrived in Mesoamerica just after the discovery of America and had an opportunity to become familiar with what was left of the ancient civilizations and to talk with old Nahuas (León Portilla, 1971). In his work the importance of chia in Aztec society is also emphasized.

In the first volume, written in 1570, Durán listed chia as one of the tributes that was paid to the Aztecs by defeated nations in order to save their lives and avoid destruction of their towns and properties. In describing the Aztec victory over the Azcaputzaleas and the lord of Texcoco, Durán stated: "The Mexicans, following their victory, were filled with anger and fury. They followed them until they put them in the woods, where the Azcaputzaleas surrendered. They promised to build houses, plough their lands, and pay a tribute to them forever. They also promised to give them stone, lime, wood, and anything they needed to survive. Almost all corn, beans, chia, chiles, and any kinds of vegetables and seeds had to be given to them" (1570:355).

In his second volume Durán referred to the Aztec calendar: "In these nations, these figures helped them to know exactly when they had to grow, to harvest, to farm and to culture the corn, to weed, to store, to thresh, to sow the beans and the chia. Order was strictly followed; for example, they knew that in a certain month they worshiped a certain god and that the day after that something else happened and so on" (1579:226).

The Codex Badianus, also known as Codex Barberini, refers to chia as well, describing its uses in pre-Columbian medicine. This codex, finished in 1552, originally was written in Nahuatl by an Indian doctor, Martín de la Cruz, and then translated into Latin and Spanish by Juan Badiano, a native from Xochimilco. This codex was discovered in the Vatican Library in 1929 and returned in May 1990 to Mexico when Pope John Paul II visited. This handwritten document is considered the most important in terms of describing Aztec medicine, since it had not been interpreted and had European explanations or comments added (Gomez Pompa, 1993).

Fray Francisco Cervantes de Salazar, a Spanish historian who studied in Spain, Flanders, and Italy, moved to Mexico in 1551 to teach Latin at the Real y Pontífica Universidad de México (Royal and Papal University of Mexico). He became the official chronicler, knew Cortés personally, and established a deep friendship with his son Martín Cortés. He is considered one of the most important humanists to write about America, and his six-volume work, *Crónica de la Nueva España* (Chronicle of New Spain), written in 1554, is considered the most valuable of all the historical accounts of the Mexican conquest. It is housed in the Biblioteca Nacional de Madrid. In the *Crónica* Cervantes de Salazar lists chia as the Aztecs' second most important crop after corn. He describes the seed, how the Indians used it, and how they sold it in the markets.

Two other valuable sources of information are the three-volume *Veinte i un libros rituales y monarquía indiana* (Twenty-one Ceremonial Books and the Indian Monarchy), written by Fray Juan de Torquemada in 1615, and the *Storia antica del Messico* (Ancient History of Mexico), written by the Jesuit priest Francisco Javier Clavijero in 1780.

Torquemada (1615) describes the first century of life in New Spain. His account is based on codices of Mexican, Telzascan, and other Mesoamerican nations as well as the traditions of natives who survived the conquest. Chia is mentioned throughout this work. Torquemada also describes different aspects of daily life, such as women participating in agriculture. In volume 2, chapter 33, he says, "Tired of running away, Necahualcoyot reached a country estate, where some peasant women were cleaning some little piles of chia (which is similar to linseed). When these women were resting they saw people coming from Maxtla." Clavijero (1780) meticulously describes the cultural evolution of the Nahua nation, including its economy, agriculture, social organization, religion, and political institutions. He refers to chia as being a highly energetic grain.

These ancient codices are important historical documents and provide valuable information. All clearly show the importance of chia in the daily life of the Aztec people and in the Nahua nations in general when the Spanish conquerors arrived.

Important Crops of the Ancient People of Mesoamerica

As stated earlier, Mesoamerica is considered one of the principal plant domestication centers of the world. Vavilov (1931) lists it as one of the eight centers from which domesticated plants spread around the world.

Ancient Mesoamericans had very few domesticated animals, but they had an impressively rich list of plants, especially compared to the list of plants that were domesticated in the Old World at that time (Benson, 1977). At the time of the conquest, Mesoamerica had at least fifty domesticated botanical species having different uses (Hawkes, 1998); among them, those listed in table 3.2 were most prominent. Four of the species stood out from a nutritional point of view: amaranth, beans, chia, and corn. These four comprised the main components of the daily diet, and the Aztecs thought of them as being equally valuable (Soustelle, 1955; Sanders, 1976; Lucena, 1992).

The extent of plants cultivated and the uses made of them by pre-Columbian people at the time of the conquest astounded European societies of that time. An example of this admiration was demonstrated by the success of the book entitled *Dos libros* (Two Books) written by a doctor, Nicolas Monardes, and published in Seville, Spain, in 1565. Later it became known as *Historia de las cosas que se traen de nuestras Indias Occidentales que sirven en medicina* (History of Things Used in Medicine Brought from Our Occidental Indians). It was reprinted in 1569 and later translated into Latin, English, French, Italian, and German and partially into Dutch. Its success had no precedent in the sixteenth century. Europeans received with even more interest Monardes's second work, published in 1571. Eventually, a compilation entitled *Primera y segunda y tercera partes de la historia medicinal de las cosas que se traen de nuestras Indias Occidentales* (First, Second, and Third Parts of the Medicinal History of Things from Our Occidental Indians) was published in 1574 (Monardes, 1574; Lozoya, 1990).

In 1569 Dr. Francisco Hernández, because of his reputation as a medical doctor and naturalist, was sent to America by Philip II to write the natural history of New Spain, with an emphasis on plants and animals having curative properties. In 1576 Hernández sent his work to Spain, where it was housed in the Biblioteca Real del Escorial. When this library was destroyed by fire in 1671 it was thought that his work was lost. However, a manuscript entitled *Materia medicinal de la Nueva España* (*Curative Material of*

TABLE 3.2. Some of the plants cultivated in Mesoamerica when
Christopher Columbus arrived

Scientific name	Common name Mexico	Common name United States
Agave spp.	Maguey	Agave
Amaranthus leucocarpus W.	Alegría	Amaranth
Arachis hypogaea L.	Cacahuate	Peanut
Canavalia ensiformis (L.) DC.	Haba blanca	Lima bean, broad bean
Capsicum annum L.	Chile	Chile
C. frutescens L.	Variedad de chile	Chile
Casimiroa edulis L.	Zapote blanco	—
Chenopodium nuttalliae S.	Huauzontle	Quinoa
Crataegus pubescens S.	Tejocote	—
Cucurbita spp.	Calabazas	Squash
Gossypium hirsutum L.[1]	Algodón	Cotton
Helianthus annus L.	Girasol	Sunflower
Ipomea batatas L.	Camote	Sweet potato
Leucaena spp.	Guaje	Leucena
Lycopersicum esculentum M.	Jitomate	Tomato
Manilkaria spp.	Nopales	Nopales
Nicotiana tabacum L.[1]	Picietl, tabaco	Tobacco
Opuntia spp.	Nopales	Nopales
Pachyrrihizus erosus L.	Jícama	Jicama
Persea americana M.	Aguacate, palta	Avocado
Phaseolus acutifolius A.	Tepary	Tepary bean
P. coccineus L.	Ayécotl, cimatl	Bean
P. vulgaris L.	Frijole, poroto	Bean
Porophyllum spp.	Quelites, verduras	Vegetables
Rumex spp.	Quelites	Vegetables
Salvia hispanica L.	Chía	Chia
Sechium edule Sw.	Chayote	—
Suaeda torreyana	Quelite salado	—
Theobroma cacao L.	Cacao	Cacao, cocoa
Zea mays L.	Maíz	Corn, maize

1. Not edible.
Sources: Sauer, 1950; Dressler, 1953; Hernández, 1985; Torres, 1985; Rojas Rabiela, 1993a.

New Spain) written by Hernández was discovered in 1999 in the Biblioteca
de la Facultad de Medicina de la Universidad Complutense de Madrid. The
content of this recently discovered work confirms the extensive knowledge
and utilization of plants that the Aztecs practiced.

The respect and interest that the pre-Columbian Nahuas had for plants
and animals are demonstrated by the botanical gardens and zoos developed in different locations throughout their territory. Europeans had not

yet even thought of building such things, only opening the first ones in 1543 in Padua and 1546 in Pisa, Italy (Cervantes de Salazar, 1554; Gortari, 1979; Garibay, 1989). Using the botanical gardens, Aztec doctors conducted research, practicing first on their own bodies and later using proven treatments to cure patients. When the Aztecs conquered a nation they included unknown plants among the tributes they demanded. They planted, harvested, and studied these (Gortari, 1979). Hence, the botanical gardens served ancient Mexico as true research and teaching centers, and the people used native plants as well as those introduced from other places for medical purposes.

The diet of ancient Mexicans can be classified as light. It was based on corn, which was eaten in cakes, soups, and tamales, and these were consumed along with chia, beans, and amaranth. In addition to the four main crops ancient Mexican diets included many other plants, both wild and domesticated, some insects, and often small quantities of meat from *huajolote* (turkey), *quetzalcoxcox* (pheasant), partridge, crow, *canauhtli* (duck), *mazatl* (deer), wild boar, pigeon, hare, and *tochtli* (rabbit) (Sahagún, 1579). Pre-Columbian diets were more varied than those of the people who live in the same areas today.

Five hundred years later studies have concluded that pre-Columbian diets were nutritionally superior to present-day diets (Ortiz de Montellano, 1978). It is interesting to note that a diet derived solely from the four grains consumed by the Aztecs meets today's dietary requirements as set out by the Food and Agriculture Organization and the World Health Organization (Food and Agriculture Organization, 1971; Ortiz de Montellano, 1978; MacLaren and Sugiura, 1991).

Chia's Role in Mesoamerican History

The Aztecs and Chia

There is evidence that chia seed was first used as food as early as 3500 B.C. and was a cash crop in the center of Mexico between 1500 and 900 B.C. Chia was cultivated in the Valley of Mexico between 2600 and 2000 B.C. by the Teotihuacán and Toltec civilizations and was one of the main components of the Aztec diet. Thus, chia was cropped before the Aztecs arrived in the Valley of

TABLE 3.3. Nahuatl words related to chia

Nahuatl	Spanish	English
Chiacpahtic	Muy aceitoso, muy grasoso	Very oily, very greasy
Chiactic	Aceitoso, grasoso	Oily, greasy
Chiahuacaayo	Aceitoso	Oily
Chiahuacayo	Grasoso	Greasy
Chiahuacayotl	Untuosidad	Greasiness
Chiahuac	Grasoso, grasiento, gordura, aceitoso	Fatty, greasy, fat, oily
Chiahua	Se hace grasoso, pastos, exuda materia, se vuelve grasoso, es grasa, es aceitoso, mancha	It becomes greasy, it becomes soggy, it exudes matter, it gets greasy, it is fat, it is oily, it stains
Chiahuizayo	Tiene fluidos cerosos, es grasoso	Has waxy fluids, is greasy
Chiahuiztli	Humor, grasa	Humor, grease
Chiancaca	Mazapán	Marzipan
Chian	Chía	Chia
Chiane	Propietario de chía	One who owns chia
Chianio	Tener chía	Having chia
Chiantzotzolatolli	Atole de chía arrugada	Atole made with wrinkled chia
Chiantzotzollo	Tener chía arrugada	Having wrinkled chia
Chiantzotzol	Chan o chía arrugada	Wrinkled chia
Chianpitzaoal	Chía de semilla pequeña	Small seeded chia
Pinolatl	Bebida de maíz y chía	Drink of corn and chia
Pinolhuia	Producir pinole (pinolatl o pinolli)	Produce pinole (pinolatl or pinolli)
Pinolli	Mezcla de harina de maíz y chía	Mixture of corn flour and chia
Pinoloa	Hacer pinole (pinolatl o pinolli)	To make pinole (pinolatl or pinolli)

Source: Adapted from Wimmer, 2001.

Mexico (Rodríguez Vallejo, 1992). Of interest is the fact that the main area of natural dispersion of chia coincides with the region that is considered the probable origin of the Aztecs (Hernández, 1993; Hernández Gómez, 1994).

Pre-Columbian civilizations used chia as a raw material for making medicines, nutritional compounds, and even paints. Because of chia's many uses a number of Nahuatl words were related to chia (see table 3.3). Chia was used by the Aztecs as food, mixed with other foods, mixed in water and drunk as a beverage, ground into flour, included in medicines, fed to birds, and pressed for oil and then used as a base for face and body paints and to protect religious statues and paintings from the elements. Chia flour could be stored for many years and could be easily carried on long trips, serving as a high-energy food. The Aztecs also offered chia to the gods during religious ceremonies (Codex Mendoza, 1542; Codex Badianus, 1552; Durán, 1570; Hernández, 1575; Sahagún, 1579; Torquemada, 1615).

Cervantes de Salazar in the *Crónica de la Nueva España* summarized the many uses for chia: "Chia can be drunk and made into flour with corn, and it keeps fresh and edible. Chia grains were given to birds in cages as birdseed in Castile. Mixed with water, it can be used to polish paintings, and, spread over skin burns, it heals them very quickly" (bk. 1, chap. 6). "Feet and legs were greased with it so as not to be harmed by water" (bk. 3, chap. 19).

Chia cultivation by other contemporary Aztec nations is documented in the Codex Mendoza. It was noted in the annual tributes paid by conquered nations as well as in the descriptions made by Sahagún (1579) regarding the productive characteristics of the ecosystems inhabited by these nations. In book 10, chapter 11 Sahagún, when referring to the Quaochpnme nation, which was situated in what is now the Mexican state of Michoacán, says: "The supplies such as corn, beans, pits, and fruit and the seeds for maintenance called *huauhtli y chian* grow very well" (1579:609).

When the Aztecs conquered new territories, chia was one of the first things they brought with them. For example, when they defeated the Oztoman and Alauiztla nations they sent settlers to live in and colonize these regions and replace the people who died during the battles. Regarding this settlement process, Durán describes the benefits the new settlers received for moving: "After they were placed in those lands, parcels and houses were distributed between them, and they marked their belongings. Corn, chile peppers, beans, chia, and all other kinds of seeds and vegetables that they ate for their sustenance that year were given out to them. Everything was brought to those places under King Ahuitzotl's command so that they would have enough to eat till next year's harvest" (1579:355).

Chia as a Food. Chia seeds mixed with amaranth seeds after both had been roasted were used to produce *tzoalli*, a dough (Torquemada, 1615; Clavijero, 1780; Soustelle, 1955). This dough, mixed with black maguey syrup and sometimes with corn flour as well, was widely used in the daily diet of the Aztecs. It also had an important religious significance, as indicated by its offering during religious ceremonies (Durán, 1570; Hernández, 1575; Sahagún, 1579). Today Mexicans still produce and consume tzoalli but with changes brought about by the conquerors. Chia is no longer used, and the maguey syrup has been replaced with honey. (Bees were introduced to America after the conquest.) The Nahuatl name for the dough was replaced by the Spanish name *alegría*.

Chia flour made from roasted chia seeds was used to prepare a refreshing and nourishing drink (Sahagún, 1579; Torquemada, 1615). It is quite probable that the drink *chía fresca*, which is made today in Mexico, Arizona, and California by the descendants of the Nahuas, came from it.

Hernández describes the use of chia in a beverage he named *chianatolli* (figure 3.4): "We could deal with *chianatolli* in the same chapter as chian, but it seems to be necessary to mention it now. Among the different ways of preparing this drink, it is known that the chian seeds, slightly toasted in a *comal* and then ground and stored, kept their flavor all year long. When the powder was needed, it was mixed with water, shaken, until it got so thick that it became tasty. Some take this drink alone, and others add some chile to it" (1576:269, 270).

Hernández's statement also points out another important characteristic of chia; that is, once it was ground chia flour could be stored for months and even years before being used to prepare food. Chia flour's ability to be stored for long periods of time is an unusual characteristic for flour made from oilseeds. This quality also allowed the annual tributes of chia that were received by Tenochtitlán to be delivered in troxes of flour as well as seed. An example is that of Tlatelolco, which sent forty baskets of *chianpinolli* (chia flour) every eighty days (Codex Mendoza, 1542).

Atolli was a gruel made from vegetable flour boiled in water. The flour came from different cooked grains, generally corn, chia, or amaranth. It was named either *atolli chiampitzahuac* or *atolli chianpitzaoal* depending on whether it was made with corn or chia flour. Today the gruel made of corn is called *atole* and is still an important dish in the Mexican diet.

Iztauhiyatl was a beverage prepared using *Artemisia mexicana* W. (Wimmer, 2001) and chia flour. Hernández describes this beverage in his *Antigüedades de la Nueva España*: "They also prepare little cups of cooked *yztauhyatll* (*iztauhiyatl*), with chia flour; those who are not used to drinking this beverage find it sour and unpleasant, but those who are used to it find it very tasty" (1575:71).

Sahagún (1579) describes bars made of almonds, chia, and honey that were sold in the public markets; he refers to them using the Spanish word *turrones*. In book 9, chapter 10 of the Codex Florentino he describes the

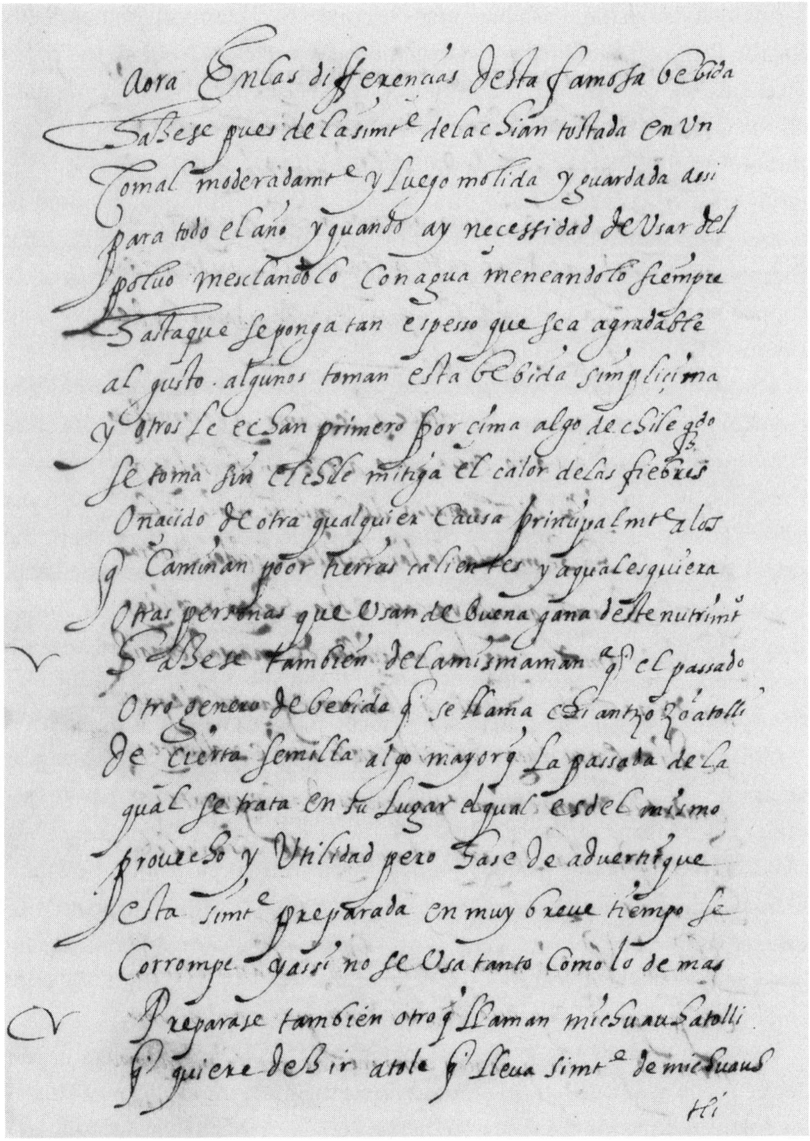

aora en las differencias desta famosa bebida
Sabese pues de la simt.e de la chian tostada en un
comal moderadamt.e y luego molida y guardada assi
para todo el año y quando ay necessidad de usar del
polvo mesclandolo con agua meneandolo siempre
hasta que se ponga tan espesso que sea agradable
al gusto. algunos toman esta bebida simplicissima
y otros le echan primero por cima algo de chile q̃do
se toma sin el chile mitiga el calor de las fiebres
o nacido de otra qualquier causa principalmt.e a los
q̃ caminan por tierras calientes y a qualesquiera
otras personas que usan de buena gana deste nutrimt.o
Hazese tambien de la misma man.a q̃ el passado
otro genero de bebida q̃ se llama chiantzoçoatolli
de cierta semilla algo mayor q̃ la passada de la
qual se trata en su lugar el qual es del mismo
provecho y utilidad pero hase de advertir que
esta simt.e preparada en muy breve tiempo se
corrompe y assi no se usa tanto como lo demas
Preparase tambien otro q̃ llaman michuauhatolli
q̃ quiere dezir atole q̃ lleva simt.e de michuauh
tli

FIGURE 3.4. Copy of page 270 of Francisco Hernández's manuscript, "Materia medicinal de la Nueva España" (Curative Material of New Spain, 1576), in which he talks about the use of chia in a beverage named *chianatolli*. (Courtesy of the Biblioteca de la Facultad de Medicina de la Universidad Complutense de Madrid.)

foods included in the lavish banquets organized by the important merchants for the Panquetzaliztli party, to which other merchants from all the provinces that comprised the Aztec Empire were invited: "And then he prepared all the grains of dried maize that would be needed. In wooden bins he put them. And the beans he also piled into wooden bins, and the wrinkled chia [and] small chia seeds. Using bins he placed about all things required to assist them, that they might not go hungry, that they might drink—that there would be what all might drink; [and] merchants' vessels in which atole topped with squash seeds might be served" (translated from the Nahuatl version by Anderson and Dibble, 1963:48).

Torquemada, who arrived in the New World just after the collapse of the Aztec Empire, describes in volume 2, book 13, chapter 23 of *Veinte i un libros rituales y monarquía indiana* parties given by Aztecs lords and points out the differences in the way chia was served to men and women: "The most important women belonging to the authorities who were invited ate to the side, with the same kind of food given to them. The main difference lay in the way they drank it, because instead of cacao (which they didn't drink) they were given *chian mazamorra*, a cold but tasty soup made of some seed, usually adding a chile mixture over it, which was called *panilli*. They ate it in the same way we eat our porridge today, with some syrup poured on top."

Chia was considered by the Aztecs to be a highly energetic grain and was an essential food during military exercises. Clavijero refers to this in volume 1 of the *Storia antica del Messico*: "The soldier who carried a small bag of corn and chia flour considered himself well stocked. Whenever he found it necessary, he poured some water on the amount of flour he wanted to eat and then added some maguey syrup. With this delicious and nourishing beverage he was able to resist the heat of the sun and the fatigue of war" (1780:54).

Durán, in volume 2, chapter 40 of *Historia de las Indias*, refers to the Aztec battle against Metztitlán, describing the great importance of chia as an energy source for the Aztec soldiers:

> The Metztitlán people had requested aid from the Huaxtecs, who, when they saw the multitude of soldiers roaring at them, stood firm and then counterattacked. In this attack three hundred of Tizoc's men were killed, which was a disaster for his army. The Aztecs, desperate and not knowing how to get out of this situation, threw a squadron of young boys into the fray. These were

eighteen- to twenty-year-old boys who always accompanied the regular army to war but just as observers in order to lose their fear of fighting in the future. They were given weapons and were ordered to attack with courage and do all that they could in order to gain the reputation of being brave warriors. These youths and the soldiers who had returned from the earlier battle to get some rest were each given a bowl of chia gruel. The youths attacked with such spirit that they captured forty soldiers from among the Metztitlán and Huaxtec warriors. When it was seen that these men had been captured, the enemy troops disbanded, and the Aztecs then forced them back across the Quetzalatl River. This had been done by the youths, who had accomplished what the regular army had failed to do. (1579:304)

Chia was a basic ingredient in a number of dishes and beverages and was widely used by the Nahuas, including during social events related to religious festivals such as *izcalli*, the ceremony in which the ears of every boy and girl born since the previous ceremony were pierced. In book 3, chapter 37 of the Codex Florentino Sahagún wrote: "And when this was done, parents looked for godfathers and godmothers, which in their language were called uncles and aunts, *tetla* and *teaui*, to hold their children when their ears were pierced; then they offered flour made from a seed called chian. The godfathers were given a tawny or bright red blanket, and the godmothers were given their *huipil*" (1579:154).

Chia as a Medicine. In Aztec society chia was also highly regarded for medicinal use. In chapter 12, book 11 of the Codex Florentino Sahagún describes the use of chia for the treatment of different illnesses, either consuming it alone or along with other medicinal herbs:

It is ground raw. A little is mixed with opossum tail [and water], just a little perhaps one-half the length of the little finger, also raw. It is also required [by] the woman who is about to give birth; she drinks it; she will promptly give birth. When it is to be drunk, it is just this alone, in preference to drinking the aforementioned ciuapatli or nopal. This chia is very good; still, few people know it. And the root of the chia is mixed with the root of the quetzalhuexotl. They are ground together; an atole is made. The chia is raw. It is required by one who spits blood, who cannot stop it, who just coughs constantly, whose blood comes from within. And it also cures a dry cough, and dislodges the flux. He is to drink it two or three times for it to be stopped. The chia is sown. It grows yearly. And this is ground raw; the juice is pressed out. It is to be drunk during fasting, for it clears the chest. Also it is like atole when mixed with grains of maize or with toasted tortillas. (Translated from Nahuatl version by Anderson and Dibble, 1963:181)

Chapter 8 of the Codex Badianus lists chia as a medicine: "When the flow of the urine is shut off, to open it take the roots of the plants mamaxtla and cohuanene-pilli, the tlatlauhqui amoxtli, the very white flower yollo-xochitl, and the tail of a sucking puppy; grind these up in acrid tasting water, macerate the well-known chian seed therein, and administer it" (1552:59; copied from the English edition by William Gates that is translated from the original Latin).

Hernández, in his *Materia medicinal de la Nueva España*, lists chia in the first part of book 3, which is dedicated to herbs that taste salty or sweet. He points out the medical uses of chia when talking about a beverage prepared from roasted ground chia: "When taken without chile, the high tempera-ture of the body—caused either by fever or by any other cause, especially for those who walk in hot climates—is relieved. This is true for anyone willing to take this nourishment" (1576:270).

In the *Nueva farmacopea de México* (New Pharmacopoeia of Mexico), published in 1874 by the Sociedad Farmacéutica de México, chia is included in the list of drugs and plants that have pharmaceutical uses (American Jour-nal of Pharmacy, 1885). Chia oil is listed as an emollient and could be intro-duced into the eye for extracting extraneous bodies, since the gelatinous mass formed when chia seeds are soaked in water helps to remove foreign materials from the eye. Chia seeds placed in water make a refreshing bev-erage for those who have a fever or are ill. This is due to the mucilage the seeds contain, and they were widely used in this manner in California and Mexico at the end of the nineteenth century. It should be noted here that the chia used in California was *Salvia columbariae*, not the *S. hispanica* that was used in Mexico. Doctors of that time also used it as a gargle and as an eye lotion (Planchon and Collin, 1895).

Chia's Other Uses. In volume 2, book 4 Torquemada (1615) described the Nahua markets and cited other uses for chia in addition to food: "And this is how attractive the markets were. Everything was placed in order and harmony. On one side the corn was sold on the cob and was called *centli* and on the other as grain. Next to these other seeds such as beans and chian, which is like *zaragotana*, were sold. Out of chian oil similar to linseed oil was made. It is spread on the feet and legs to keep them from being harmed by water. It is also used for cooking because it is healthy and tasty. Chian is ground for beverages and mixed with amaranth seeds."

Chia oil, known as *chiamatl* by the ancient Mexicans, was used as a cosmetic. Both Aztec men and women used scents and perfumes, often applied in the form of ointments (Cervantes de Salazar, 1554; Torquemada, 1615). Chia oil was a component of these ointments, presumably because of its emollient properties (J. Brown, Scottsdale, Arizona, personal communication, 1998).

Chia had a prominent use in pre-Columbian paintings, as it improved the drying qualities of paints and varnishes. The varnishes made with chia oil have two distinct characteristics: they do not yellow with time, and the clarity and transparency are exceptional. Chia oil also imparts a shine to colors when used in paints (Clavijero, 1780; Rulfo, 1937; Soustelle, 1955). The individuals who accompanied the Spanish conquerors and wrote the sixteenth-century codices used native artists to illustrate them with paints based on chia oil. Even after five centuries the illustrations in these manuscripts, such as in the 1579 Codex Florentino, are unsurpassed for their brilliant colors and clarity (United States Department of Agriculture, 1943). In book 3, chapter 19 Cervantes de Salazar (1554) pointed out the notable characteristics of chia oil when used for paintings: "The chia oil is so good that, spread on a painting, it keeps its vividness and protects the painting's colors against air and water."

The protective action that chia oil imparted to Aztec paintings reminded the conquerors of the protection given by flaxseed oil, which was used in the Old World. Fray Alonso de la Rea spoke of his admiration for chia oil in his 1643 *Crónica de la orden de N. Seráfico P. S. Francisco, provincia de S. Pedro y S. Pablo de Mechoacán en la Nueva España* (Chronicles of the [Holy] Order of the N. Seráfico P. S. Francisco, Province of Saint Peter and Saint Paul of Michoacán in New Spain): "The paint of Periban, which has so far not been imitated, was invented in this province. Apart from being bright, the varnish is so strong that it will not be affected by the passing of time. It is natural for all colors to fade with the passing of time. Warm water, washing, and rubbing loosen them, but the colors of Michoacán are not affected nor faded with time, becoming as much a part of the wood or vase, lasting the same length of time."

Fray Pablo de la Purísima Concepción Beaumont, a professor of anatomy and surgery at the Royal Hospital of Mexico, remarked how the paintings made by the Tarascos, who were the ancient inhabitants of the present state of Michoacán, were preserved because of the use of chia oil. In his 1792 work, *Crónica de Mechoacán*, Beaumont said: "These Tarascos are the first inventors of the paint that has so far not been imitated in wooden objects. This paint can still be appreciated in basins of Periban and in what today is being worked on in Coupao. It is so durable that put together with the same carved piece its duration and permanence are remarkable."

In Guatemala during colonial times chia oil was also used in paints, and growing it as a crop was a good business. This was noted in a 1787 report written by the archbishop of Guatemala, who referred to his visit to San Pedro de la Laguna by saying, "There is a large harvest of beans of beautiful quality and chian. They obtain quite a lot of money from them, and they are used for drinks and by painters" (Cortéz y Larraz, 1958:bk. 1, vol. 20, p. 96).

Hernández describes the Texcoco and Tenochtitlán markets as he viewed them fifty years after the fall of the Aztec Empire. He pointed out the commercialization and utilization not only of chia seed but of chia oil as well and described two very different uses for it: "They also sell chia oil, used to preserve the gods' statues from the erosion of water and weather, and to season food" (Hernández, 1575:106).

Today's painters know about the high quality of chia oil and consider it superior to linseed or flaxseed oil (Hernández Gómez, 1994; Heil, 1995; Niblo, 1995). The superiority of chia oil over flax oil is due to the higher concentration of linolenic acid. This fatty acid is fundamental to paint quality because it favors fast oxygenation, speeding the drying process and increasing the long-lasting stability of the colors. The advantage that chia oil has over linseed oil was confirmed during the last century by a 1918 patent obtained on a process to produce a drying oil from chia (Baughman and Jamieson, 1929).

Today chia oil is still used by craftsmen in the Mexican states of Chiapas, Guerrero, and Michoacán and in Mexico City when preparing lacquers, locally known as *maque*, to paint *jicaras* (*Crescentia* spp.), *guajes* (*Lajenaria* sp.), and other native flora used in various crafts. Maque art flourished in ancient Mexico long before the Spanish arrived. How the pre-Columbian nations developed such a sophisticated art is still a mystery.

The Asociación Mexicana de Arte y Cultura Popular (AMACUP), with headquarters in Mexico City, makes extensive use of chia oil in its well-known Indian handicrafts, primarily through artisans living in the southern state of Chiapas. According to Marta Turok, founder and director of AMACUP, chia is one of the reasons for the success of the handicrafts produced. The glossy lacquer finish is obtained using the traditional process and chia oil and creates finishes in warm chocolate browns, forest greens, and blood reds (Masuoka, 2001).

C. Heil describes the system used by Mexican artisans to extract chia oil: "Chia oil is extracted by slowly roasting the seeds on a flat metal or clay dish on a low fire until they are uniformly light brown, or the seeds begin to pop open. When cool, the seeds are ground in a hand-mill or on a stone pestle. Hot water is added to the fine flour to form a mushy paste, which, when cool, is kneaded for about an hour or until the oil begins to drip. The paste is wrapped in a cloth and twisted to wring out the oil. Finally, the oil is boiled to preserve it until it is needed" (1995:4).

At the end of the twentieth century the demand for Mexican handicrafts that used lacquer or shellac increased remarkably. Because of inadequate supplies of chia oil and shellac the artisans began to use flaxseed oil and automotive lacquer as substitutes. This decreased the quality of the finished product dramatically. Worried about decreasing quality, the Cultural Bancomer Foundation, a nonprofit organization created by the Bank of Mexico, promoted a series of meetings among artisans from different Mexican states to discuss the issue. The attendees, along with the Cultural Bancomer Foundation, agreed to find ways of getting the correct raw materials to the centers that lacked them in order to preserve the quality of the goods produced.

The Maya and Chia

Chiapas, which is located within what was ancient Mayan territory, derives its name from the Nahuatl words *chia* and *apan*, which means "in or on the water." Hence, Chiapan means chia river or chia water. The city of Chiapas was founded on the banks of the Río Grijalva by a group that probably came from Central America during the sixth century. These people were called

Chiapas or Chiapanecas and were known as Napinioka in the Chiapaneca language.

We have not found evidence that chia was cultivated by the Maya at the height of their civilization, that is, between 800 B.C. and A.D. 900. There is evidence, however, of intense commerce between Teotihuacán and the Maya over several centuries. This makes it impossible to believe that chia was unknown to this extraordinary civilization, which occupied a large part of Mexico, Guatemala, Honduras, and El Salvador.

Despite the assumption made by some archaeologists, Nahuas were probably not present in the Mayan region during the Classic period (200 B.C.–A.D. 900); instead, they arrived during the post-Classic period following the consolidation of the Aztec Empire as the center of power (Christensen, 1996). This could explain why chia was not cultivated by the Mayan civilization during its age of splendor; instead, the practice started after the Maya abandoned their cities.

Don Diego García de Palacio, in a letter sent in 1583 to the king of Spain, refers to chia as a food of the Indians living in what is now Guatemala. García de Palacio was an *oydor* (listener) of the Real Audiencia de Guatemala and was commanded to visit a number of Guatemalan provinces and report upon them. He described the ancient provinces of Guazaapan, Izalco, Cuscatlán, and Chiquimula by giving an account of the language, customs, and religion of the natives along with a description of the famous ruins of Copan in Honduras. He described a ceremony of the Chontales natives that included "a round stone idol called Ycelaca, with two faces, one on the front and one on the back, with many eyes. It was said that he was the god that knew the present and the past and that he could see everything. He had both faces and eyes covered with blood. Deer, hens, rabbits, bell pepper, chian, and lots of other products they used in those days were sacrificed to him" (García de Palacio, 1583:132).

Today in the Chiapas region of Mexico, where the ruins of the impressive Mayan city of Palenque were discovered in 1840, are found two beverages known as *pozol* and *tazcalate* in the Chiapaneca language. In Spanish, tazcalate is known as *agua de chía* (chia water). The first drink is based on corn and the second on chia. These are taken at noon as a refreshment when conditions of high temperature and humidity exist.

Surviving the Conquerors' Colonization

The Spanish conquest repressed the natives, suppressed their traditions, and destroyed most of the intensive agricultural production and commercialization system that had existed. Many crops that had held a major position in pre-Columbian American diets were banned by the Spanish because of their close association with religion. They were replaced by foreign species (wheat, barley, rice, etc.) that were in demand by the conquerors (Soustelle, 1955; Engel, 1987).

In chapter 10 of his 1568 work *La verdadera historia de la conquista de México* (The True History of the Conquest of Mexico), which was translated into English by Maurice Keatinge and edited by J. Wright and John Dead in 1800, Bernal Díaz del Castillo refers to the changes that took place in Nahua agriculture following the Spanish conquest: "Advantages resulting from the conquest. Concluding observations of the author . . . tilling of land as was done before our arrival; and now they rear flock, and break bullocks, and plow, sow wheat, manure, reap, fell, and make bread and biscuits. They have planted their lands and inheritances with the fruit trees of Old Spain, harvested the fruit, cut down the unwholesome peach trees, and pulled out the plantains, to make room for quince, apple, and pear trees, which they hold in high esteem."

As part of the evangelization process, the friars ordered the destruction of pre-Hispanic temples and then used the stones to build churches and monasteries. This radical methodology was used not only with "heathen" temples but also with every custom related to pre-Hispanic religions. As a consequence, many crops that had held honored positions in native cultures for thousands of years were deliberately eliminated.

Of the four basic crops in the Aztec diet, only chia and amaranth lost their privileged places and almost disappeared. To understand the scope of the conquerors' persecution of chia and amaranth it is necessary to describe some of the fundamental relationships between the Catholic faith and the Aztec religion. One similarity that strongly influenced the Spanish to stop the growing and use of these two crops was the Aztec custom of cutting images of gods made from dough into pieces and then eating them at the end of religious ceremonies. This custom, and its similarity to Catholic Communion, horrified the friars.

Durán (1570) wrote an entire book describing Aztec religious ceremonies, with two chapters devoted to the god Huitzilopochtli. The importance that the religious ceremonies for the god Huitzilopochtli had in the Aztec nation, combined with human sacrifices, gave the conquerors great concern and makes it necessary to summarize part of the work of Durán here. This should help explain why the tremendous decrease in chia production took place following the discovery of America.

The Aztec ceremony to honor the god Huitzilopochtli started at the end of sunrise on a day in April, with the date varying by eight to ten days. Many times the date coincided with Easter. From noon of the day prior to the ceremony the Aztecs did not eat anything except tzoalli with syrup and did not drink anything, not even water. This fasting continued until the end of the ceremony. For the ceremony tzoalli was used to build models of the god Huitzilopochtli. The models were about the same size as a human and were in a classic squatting position. These were shown to each individual who was going to be sacrificed, with the person being told, "This is your god." Before the sacrifice took place maidens devoted to the god brought numerous bone-shaped pieces made from tzoalli and gave them to young men, also devoted to the god, who deposited them around the idol. After the sacrifice the priests spread the captive's blood over the idol and then cut not only the bone-shaped pieces but the idol as well into numerous pieces. Next, starting from the oldest man, all of the people, including children, were fed the pieces. They received them with great devotion and admiration because they felt they were eating the flesh and bones of the god, of whom they were unworthy. People who knew a sick person asked for a piece and took it to that person with great reverence and veneration. Everyone who took part in this ceremony was required to give a tithe to the Aztec state, the king, and the priests. This tithe had to be paid with chia seed, which was then used to prepare the dough from which the idol and bones were made. This brings forth another similarity between the Aztec religion and Christianity, as Christians of that time also were required to give one tenth of their belongings to help support the Catholic Church. After finishing the ceremony the most prestigious priest, generally the oldest, went to the altar and preached, reminding the people of the ten commandments. These are essentially the same as those observed by Christians.

The many commonalities between Huitzilopochtli's ceremony and aspects of the Catholic faith not only made the Spanish conquerors think about the existence of previous contacts between both worlds but also horrified them. Hence, they denounced the ceremony as being terrible heresy (Sahagún, 1579; Durán, 1570; Solís, 1770). Although we found no sources in which the Spanish government decreed the need to eliminate the production and use of chia, we did find a number of references that discuss the need to eradicate everything that was related to pre-Columbian religions. An example of this was written by Sahagún in book 10 of the Codex Florentino under the title "Relación del autor digna de ser notada" (Narrative of the Author Deserving to Be Noted): "It was necessary to destroy all idolatrous things, every idolatrous building and even any custom that had to do with idolatrous rituals or ceremonies. This kind of belief and ceremony was present in almost every custom in the ruling republic, and that was why it was necessary to destroy them all and use police who were not contaminated by idolatry" (1579:579).

The disdain felt by the Spanish conquerors for the customs of the ancient Mexicans is clearly shown in the colloquial expression "me importa un bledo" [I don't care at all]. The word *bledo* (wild amaranth) when used as a colloquialism means something insignificant, having no importance or interest. This unfair meaning is still in use in both Spain and Hispanic America. When Fidel Castro visited Argentina on 26 May 2003 he made a speech at the University of Buenos Aires. When referring to people who criticize the government of Cuba, he said, "Me importa un bledo lo que digan de nosotros" [I don't care anything about what people say about us].

The effects of the Spanish persecution of the Aztec religion were greater on chia than on amaranth. Amaranth, known as *kiwicha* in Quechua and *qmasa* in Aymara, was one of the main crops of the Inca Empire, a sophisticated South American civilization and a contemporary of the Aztecs. Parallel development of the crop in two locations undoubtedly increased the survival of amaranth compared to chia (National Research Council, 1989).

Another factor that helped corn, beans, and amaranth but not chia to survive is the difference in their photoperiod requirements. Corn, beans, and amaranth are insensitive (or at least are not very sensitive) to a particular photoperiod and can flower in Spain and other European countries. This is not the case with chia, as it requires short days for flowering, and these are only reached in European countries when frost has killed or soon will kill the plants. Hence, this physiological requirement prevented chia from being grown in the Old World. The failure of many American plant species to adapt to European ecosystems was recognized by Clavijero: "The things from Europe work better in America than the things from America that don't work so well in Europe" (1780).

Chia managed to survive extinction as a crop following the arrival of the Spanish conquerors because of the conservation of some pre-Columbian traditions by small groups of people who were descendants of the Nahua nations. They overcame the conquerors and the cultural pressures put on them by remaining isolated in southwestern Mexico and the mountains of Guatemala. Today Nahua and Mayan descendants use this ancient grain in a popular beverage called chía fresca; however, its preparation is not like the one used by ancient Mexicans. Today chia seeds are mixed in lemonade, and this drink is consumed not only in Mexico but in Guatemala, El Salvador, Nicaragua, and the southwestern United States (New Mexico, California, and Arizona) as well.

Although chia did survive, it was cultivated in only a few locations in Mexico and in Guatemala only along the border with Mexico. El Salvador and Nicaragua retained the tradition of drinking a beverage made with chia, but the seeds are harvested from wild populations found in fields planted to other crops or on the shoulders of roads. Differences among countries in terms of chia production could be related to the still mysterious collapse of the Mayan civilization and the disappearance of most Mayan customs before the Spanish conquerors arrived. It is clear that chia's use as food by these people was less important than among the Nahua nations. This could mean that chia never was cropped by the Maya or that the cropping practices were lost due to the longer period of time that passed from when the Maya disappeared compared to that of the Aztecs.

In the southwestern United States and northwestern Mexico chia (*S. columbariae* and/or *S. carduacea*) was not cultivated but rather was collected from wild populations. Here the Spanish influence was comparatively less than on the Nahua nations. Ancient peoples of these arid regions depended heavily on chia as a staple food. Today it is used regularly by the descendants of the early people who discovered its usefulness (Hicks, 1966).

As is described in more detail in chapter 4, chia in California, Arizona, Baja California, and Sonora refers to the species *S. columbariae* B. The subject of this book, *S. hispanica* L., is not adapted to the ecosystems in those regions.

The Awakening of a Sleeping Crop

Two references that mention natives growing chia after the conquest are dated 1581 and 1585. The former is a document commanded by the king of Spain and written by Juan González, *corregidor* of Xonotla, Mexico, that was certified in the presence of the notary Marcos de Berrearce. This document, known as the *Relación de Xonotla*, is held by the Archivo General de Indias in Seville, Spain. The second is described by Teresa Rojas Rabiela (1993a), who found it while studying the history of agriculture on chinampas from pre-Hispanic times to the end of the twentieth century. The item was a report on Xochimilco written in 1585 by Fray Antonio de Ciudad Real and published in 1976 by the Universidad Autónoma de México. The first document reports chia as a crop in the Xonotla area, and the second describes chia as being one of the main crops cultivated on chinampas.

A document written in 1689 by Fray Francisco de Zuaza describes the convents in Guatemala belonging to the Franciscans. Chia is mentioned in a description of the convent of San Francisco de Panahachel: "It is located on the banks of Atitán Lake. It is a small bay or cove between two pieces of land, in an extended plain with the most fertile soil to grow all kinds of crops. This is why there is a great variety of legumes and vegetables, anise, chian, garlic, and other species as well as fruit trees from both hot and cold lands" (Zuaza, 1689:96).

Two later references about chia are dated 1780 and 1787. The first, which was a census, shows chia among the crops cultivated in San Antonio Palopó, Department of Sololá (Cortéz y Larraz, 1958; Instituto Geográfico Nacional, 2002). In the second the archbishop of Guatemala, don Pedro Cortés y Larraz, describes a chia harvest in San Pedro de la Laguna on the banks of the Atitán lagoon.

In 1874 the *Nueva farmacopea de México* reported chia as a crop being cultivated in the central high plateau as well as in other locations in Mexico (American Journal of Pharmacy, 1885). Charles Saunders (1920) noted the sale of chia in various Mexican markets. In 1929 in the state of Morelos, Mexico, Margaret Redfield listed agua de chía as a typical food in Tepoztlán, a town inhabited almost exclusively by pure natives. Both of these citations from the 1920s indicate that chia had to have been grown somewhere in the country at that time. Chia is listed as a crop in the Department of Agriculture statistics published by the Mexican Secretary of Agriculture and Promotion from 1932 to 1935 (Rulfo, 1937). According to Rulfo (1937), the Mexican government only began to record chia production in 1932, although the crop had been produced for several prior years.

Table 3.4 lists the state and the production for that state between 1932 and 1935. All of these areas are between 1,000 and 2,000 meters above sea level, most of them in the region called the Mexican High Plateau (Altiplano Mexicano). During these years the greatest production was in the state of Jalisco, with 78, 71, 92, and 88 percent of the seed produced in the municipalities of Acatic and Tepatitlán in the Jalisco Highlands (Los Altos de Jalisco). This area coincides with Aztlán, the region where the Aztec nation is thought to have originated (Rulfo, 1937; Matos Moctezuma, 1994).

In the 1990s small plots of chia were grown along with corn in the mountainous regions of Temalacacingo, Chiepetlán, and Tlalapa in the state of Guerrero; San Mateo Cautepec in the state of Puebla; Zapotlanejo and Acatic in Jalisco; and in a few locations in Morelos (Hernández Gómez, 1994; INIFAP, 1995). In 1993 Ricardo Ayerza Jr. interviewed twelve chia growers from the municipality of Acatic, Jalisco. The parents and grandparents of these individuals had lived in the region since before the nineteenth century. Table 3.5 was prepared from the data he gathered. Although reliable numbers for only 1989 through 1992 were obtained, they established the extent of chia cropping at the time. In 1993 450 hectares were planted to chia in the Los Altos de Jalisco region of Acatic County. This caused prices to fall below production costs (J. de Rosas, Acatic, Jalisco, Mexico, personal communication, 1993). The result was that growers reduced the area planted in subsequent years to less than 350 hectares.

Today in remote areas of Guatemala it is still possible to find small plots of chia cultivated by descendants of the Maya. Although the Guatemalan government reports chia as being one of its agricultural crops, it is considered a low priority for the country (Martínez Arevalo, 1996).

Chia survived more than five hundred years by remaining far from the centers of power. However, in doing so it lost much more than it gained. Among the losses are lost varieties and lost uses. The absolutely marginal position that chia held during the last five hundred years impeded the growers' ability to mechanize production and in many cases even prevented

TABLE 3.4. Mexican chia production, 1932–35

State	Area (ha)				Yield (kg/ha)				Total production (t)			
	1932	1933	1934	1935	1932	1933	1934	1935	1932	1933	1934	1935
Zacatecas	2	—	—	—	600	—	—	—	1.2	—	—	—
Chiapas	—	1	1	—	—	450	800	—	—	0.45	0.8	—
Guerrero	—	5	—	—	—	500	—	—	—	2.5	—	—
Oaxaca	—	2	2	3	277	290	380	350	—	0.58	0.76	1.05
Jalisco	26	30	70	75	493	417	600	493	12.8	12.5	42	37
Michoacán	2	2	2	7	300	320	400	300	0.6	0.64	0.8	2.1
Puebla	8	4	3	8	240	200	420	200	1.9	0.8	1.26	1.6
Total	38	44	78	93	—	—	—	—	16.5	17.5	45.6	41.8

Source: Adapted from Rulfo, 1937.

TABLE 3.5. Average area, by grower, sown to chia in
Acatic County, Jalisco, Mexico

Farmer	1992	1991	1990	1989	Average[1]
			ha		
A	15	15	—	20	16.7
B	4	—	—	—	4
C	2	—	—	—	2
D	5	3	—	—	4
E	12	21	4	—	12.3
F	5	8	5	—	6
G	2	4	2	2	2.5
H	5	—	—	—	5
I	5	7	3	—	5
J	2	2	2	—	2
K	—	5	3	—	4
L	15	15	9	9	12
M	3	6	—	—	4.5
Total	75	86	28	31	55
Average	6.3	9.6	4.76	10.3	—

1. Average over the producing years.

them from maintaining the hand processes that had been previously used. The genetic degradation that probably took place because farmers had to multiply a population composed of a mixture of varieties selected before the sixteenth century led to a nonuniformity that modern markets dislike in crops, making chia commercially nonviable.

The growers from the municipality of Acatic are truly the custodians of the Nahua chia traditions, having transmitted from generation to generation the basic knowledge of chia as a crop and saving it from disappearing. As a consequence, they have provided humanity with an opportunity to correct the misdeeds committed more than five hundred years ago by the Spanish conquerors.

Chia arrived in the twenty-first century without having incorporated the changes needed to adapt it to modern production. It has gone no further than only surviving as a raw material for making an ancestral beverage that is consumed by a few ethnic groups. Chia did not travel the same way its ancient mates such as corn, beans, tomatoes, and cocoa did; hence, it is not one of the constituents of modern human diets as the others are.

The Northwestern Argentina Regional Project (Ayerza and Coates, 1996) began in 1991 with an agreement between Partners of the Americas, Inc., a nonprofit organization located in Washington, D.C., and a group of farmers, mainly tobacco growers, from northwestern Argentina. This cooperation was orchestrated through the Farmer to Farmer Program, which was established by the U.S. Congress as part of the 1990–95 Farm Bill. The objective of the project was to identify and put into commercial production new crops that could help diversify agricultural production and increase the income of northwestern Argentina farmers. Subsequently, the University of Arizona, the University of California, the National University of Catamarca, the Rural Group Pulares, and the government of the province of Salta joined the project. In 1995 four farming organizations in the region— the CREA Los Lapachos growers group, the Jujuy and Salta Independent Sugar Cane Growers Association, the Jujuy Tobacco Growers Cooperative, and the Jujuy Chamber of Tobacco Growers—also joined.

University faculty and technical personnel have been involved in establishing research plots, providing on-farm technical advice, conducting workshops, and presenting conferences and seminars for growers during the course of the project. For example, during 1995 twelve topics were the subject of a series of workshops, conferences, and seminars held at various locations in northwestern Argentina. Seventeen scientists, growers, and company managers were brought from the United States to Argentina to provide technical assistance. Their areas of expertise included agronomy, genetics, plant physiology, mechanization, processing, economics, and marketing.

The research plots as well as demonstration plantings were located on private farms, directly involving the farming public in the project. Tests were conducted in four provinces (Catamarca, Jujuy, Salta, and Tucumán), providing wide public exposure. Seven species were identified that appeared to hold significant potential for the region. These were chia, lesquerella (*Lesquerella fendleri*), vernonia (*Vernonia galamensis*), and chan (*Hyptis suaveolens* L.), all of which are sources of industrial and edible oils; guayule (*Parthenium argentatum* G.), a source of rubber, resins, and latex; kenaf (*Hibiscus cannabinus* L.), a raw material for paper and newsprint; and doca (*Morrenia odorata*), a source of hypoallergenic fiber to make pillows, com-

TABLE 3.6. Number of growers and area commercially sown to
chia in Argentina and Bolivia

Year	Location	Province	Growers (no.)	Area planted (ha)	Average size (ha)	Yearly total (t)
	Argentina					
1992	C. del Valle	Catamarca	1	14	14	14
1993	C. del Valle	Catamarca	1	70	70	74
	Alberdi	Tucumán	1	4	4	
1994	C. del Valle	Catamarca	2	3	1.5	31
	Sumalao	Catamarca	1	20	20	
	Alberdi	Tucumán	1	5	5	
	Valle de Lerma	Salta	1	3	3	
1995	C. del Valle	Catamarca	2	3	1.5	58
	Alberdi	Tucumán	1	5	5	
	Valle de Lerma	Salta	5	40	8	
	Metan	Salta	1	10	10	
1996	Valle de Lerma	Salta	6	120	20	145
	Guemes	Salta	1	5	5	
	Perico	Jujuy	2	20	10	
1997	Valle de Lerma	Salta	3	83	27.6	48
1998	Valle de Lerma	Salta	3	107	35.6	55
1999	Valle de Lerma	Salta	12	426	35.5	255
2000	All areas	Salta	—	887	—	296
2001	All areas	Salta	—	70	—	56
	Bolivia					
1999	Santa Cruz	Santa Cruz	2	33	16.5	14
2000	Santa Cruz	Santa Cruz	1	180	180	119

forters, and other products. The most promising species identified during
the course of the project was chia, with chia being the only one commercially grown to date (Coates and Ayerza, 1996). Table 3.6 lists the sites and
number of growers involved over the life of the project and shows the evolution of this crop in Argentina and Bolivia from 1992 up to and including
its early commercial production.

Commercial yields of chia varied from year to year and from location to
location due to a number of factors, including cultural practices, climate,
weed infestations, and harvesting techniques. Cultural practices purposely
were not standardized across farms, as it was the intent of the project to
allow farmers to use those cultural practices to grow chia with which they

were familiar while providing them with general guidance as to how best to produce the crop.

The migration of the crop north from Catamarca to the province of Salta, where today production is concentrated, took place principally because of climatic conditions. In particular, frost was a factor. In Valle de Lerma frosts occur when the growth cycle has completed. The risk of losing the crop due to early frosts is low (<10 percent) compared with Catamarca and Tucumán, where frosts are generally earlier.

The Northwestern Argentina Regional Project introduced chia into Colombia and Peru as well, although it was only commercially grown there for a few years. Although chia reached an adequate level of development in the Valle del Cauca, Colombia, strong tropical rains at harvest made it difficult to combine. In Ica, which is located on the Peruvian coastal desert south of Lima, high production costs, especially for irrigation water, elevated the price beyond what the market was willing to pay. Hence, these areas were abandoned.

Subsequently, work began to market products enriched with omega-3 fatty acids using chia. Different organizations have been involved in this aspect of the project: International Flora Technologies, Inc., Gilbert, Arizona; Rural Group Pulares, Pulares, Salta, Argentina; the University of Arizona, Tucson; and the U.S. Agency for International Development (Coates and Ayerza, 1996). Currently, the scientific and technological development of chia is being undertaken by University of Arizona researchers, while the agricultural production is done by growers from Argentina and Bolivia. The research and development activities include chia adaptation to modern agriculture, determination of production areas, agricultural machinery requirements for each stage of crop production, seed cleaning and storage, cultivar selection, and product development and commercialization.

FOUR

The Renaissance of Chia

The Nahua System of Botanical Classification

The Nahua system of botanical classification identified plant groups by their fruits, roots, stems, flowers, and use. Plant names were formed in three parts that indicate plant qualities (sizes and parts), plant uses, and type of soil where grown. These terms were used in very clear and descriptive ways; however, in some cases the Nahuas formed even more complex names (Gortari, 1979). Three example names from this system are *tonalchichicaquilitl*, meaning "edible herb that grows with sun and water," *tepehoilacapitzxochitl*, "hairy flower with an arboreal stem," and *tepehoilacapitzxochitl*, "ornamental plant that grows in the hills, has a knotty stem, crawls but later turns straight and thin" (Gortari, 1979; Estrada Lugo, 1989). Table 4.1 shows part of the Nahua botanical classification system that was in use when the Spaniards arrived in America.

The Nahua botanical system was not only accurate but also extremely practical and very didactical. As both Estrada Lugo (1989) and Torres (1985) explained, due to the agglutinative (one or more words or parts of words joined to generate a new word) and metaphoric characteristics of the Nahuatl language, one word was permitted to have more than one meaning.

TABLE 4.1. Nahua taxonomic system

Plant sizes	Xihuitl	Herbs
	Quaxihitl/cuacuhtzin	Shrubs
	Quauitl	Trees
Plant parts	Tzocuit	Roots in general
	cimatl	Main tap root
	cicimatl	Main branched root
	camohtli	Tube-shaped root
	xicama	Globular root
	Tlacotl	Branch
	Cocohtli	Empty stem
	Acatl	Cane
	Quiyotl	Trunk
	Tlaxitlepeualli	Bark
	Tlapalli	Leaves in general
	atlapalli	Leaves of tree
	Xochitl	Flowers
	xochiatlapalli	Petals
	Xochicualli	Fruits
	hu chtli	Seeds
	Huitztli	Thistle
Plant uses	Quilitl	For food
	Patli	Medicinals/poison/stimulant
	Tzcatlo	Grasses
	Xichuitl	Animal food
Type of soil	Atl/ate/a	Water plants
where grown	Atlentilla	On water shores
	Aztecatl	In quiet waters
	Apantli	In irrigation ditches
	Atlan	Close to the water
	Tlalli	In land
	Tetla	In stones
	Tepetla	In hills
	Texcal	In cliffs
Color	Tliltic	Black
	Chichiltic	Red
	Istac	White
	Tlapolli	Varied colors
Other	Chichic	Bitter
	Xocotl	Sour
	Acoco	Empty
	Nacatl	Pulpy
	Tzapotl	Sweet

Sources: Gortari, 1979; Estrada Lugo, 1989.

Which Is the "Real" Chia Species?

The Nahua name *chian* referred to the chia plant, with suffixes added to describe a characteristic. For instance, *chianpitzaoal* means small chia, and *chiantzotzol* refers to wrinkled chia (Wimmer, 2001). The word *chía* is a Spanish adaptation of the Nahua word *chian* or *chien* (plural) (Watson, 1938). Some of the first people to arrive with the Spanish conquerors, such as the Franciscan friar Toribio de Benavente (1541), referred to chia as *chiyan*. In many passages of the Spanish version of the Codex Florentino Sahagún (1579) used chia and chian interchangeably. In the Nahuatl version variations also exist, as Sahagún refers to this species as chian and chien. Anderson and Dibble (1963) in their English translation of the Nahuatl version of the Codex Florentino used the word *chia* for both chian and chien; for example, "no yoan in chien, iztac chien, tliltic chien, chiantzotzol," "and also chia, white chia, black chia, wrinkled chia" (bk. 2, chap. 23, p. 65); "auh in ontlaquaque: aocmo cacaoatl in quinmacaia, ça atulli chianpitzaoac, puchtecaio caxitl, inic quinmacaia tiçatica tlacujlollo," "and when they ate, they served them no chocolate, but only atole with chia" (bk. 9, chap. 9, p. 41).

The chia that was grown by the Nahuas when Columbus arrived in America and that is now commercially grown in Argentina, Bolivia, and Mexico is *Salvia hispanica* L. During the twentieth century all of the chia that was studied was acquired from Mexican markets (Baughman and Jamieson, 1929; Rulfo, 1937; Palma, Donde, and Lloyd, 1947; Eckey, 1954; Hernández Gómez, 1994) and health food stores in Southern California (Taga, Miller, and Pratt, 1984) and is *S. hispanica* L. Chia also is the common name for a number of other plants native to Mexico and the United States. Although most belong to the genus *Salvia* (Lamiaceae), some belong to the genus *Hyptis* (Lamiaceae) and one to the genus *Amaranthus* (Amaranthaceae) (table 4.2). The fatty acid composition of several of these species is shown in table 4.3. Today, use of the name chia to denote different species of the same genus as well as plants from different genera such as *Hyptis* and *Amaranthus* could be due to the post-Columbus confusion that occurred when the Nahua botanical classification was abandoned.

TABLE 4.2. Chia species: common and scientific names

Common name	Scientific name
Chía	*Salvia hispanica* L.
Chía	*S. polystachya* O.
Chía	*S. carduacea* L.
Chía	*S. lanceolata* B.
Chía azul grande	*S. cyanea* B.
Chía cimarrona	*S. angustifolia* C.
Chía cimarrona	*S. privoides* B.
Chía cimarrona	*S. tiliaefolia* V.
Chía cimarrona	*S. dugesii* F.
Chía de campo	*S. columbariae* B.
Chía de California	*S. columbariae* B.
Chian/chiyant	*S. hispanica* L.
Chía de Colima	*Hyptis suaveolens* L.
Chía gorda	*H. suaveolens* L.
Chía grande	*H. suaveolens* L.
Chía de chapata	*Amaranthus leucocarpus* W.

S. hispanica L. and *Hyptis suaveolens* L.

A common mistake in contemporary literature is use of the word *chia* for two botanical species: *S. hispanica* L. and *Hyptis suaveolens* L. Because of this many people think that the name *chia* was used for both species by the Aztecs, as both were oil crops and the Aztecs did not distinguish between them. However, an analysis of sixteenth-century books shows this not to be the case.

Sahagún's Spanish version of the Codex Florentino shows that the Nahuas clearly differentiated between chian (*S. hispanica* L.) and another oily species named *chiantzotzotl* (*H. suaveolens* L.): "They add chia or wrinkled chia to it. It is drunk; an atole is made" (bk. 11, par. 45, Anderson and Dibble, 1963:151). In book 10, chapters 18 and 20 Sahagún referred to different kinds of traders and the goods sold by each. He pointed out that *chiantzotzotl* (plural: *chientzotzol*) and chian were sold by completely different traders:

[C]hiennamacac: ca chiane. In chiennamacac, qujnamaca in itzac chien, in aiauhchien, in coçlli, in chiencoçolli. In tlaueliloc chiennamacac: qujnamaca in chian, qujmotlatlia, itlan caquja in polocatl, in chianpolocatl, in coçolli. . . .

TABLE 4.3. Oil content and composition of some chia species

Species	Oil	Fatty acids (%)					Source
		Palmitic	Stearic	Oleic	Linoleic	Linolenic	
Salvia hispanica L.	37.4	6.3	3.1	7.8	20.2	63	Ayerza, 1995
S. polystachya O.	29.8	27	12	21	12.8	15	Bushway, Belya, and Bushway, 1981
S. carduacea B.	30	9.3	2.8	34	19	32	Hagemann, Earle, and Wolff, 1968
S. columbariae B.	32	5.8	2.8	8.9	17	6.5	Hagemann, Earle, and Wolff, 1968.
Hyptis suaveolens L.	12	8.9	1.8	8.6	80.4	0.3	Coates and Ayerza, 1995
Amaranthus leucocarpus W.	3	20	3.9	31	50.7	1	Ucciani, 1995

Chientzotzolnamacac: in chientzotzolnamacac: chieme, chienmille, chientzo-
tzole, tlamatiloani, tlaiectiani, nononqua quinamaca in chontalcaiotl, in ozo-
toman uitz, in tlaluiccaiotl, in itziocaiutl.

The chia seller is one who owns chia. The chia seller sells white chia, blighted
chia, the shriveled seeds. The bad chia seller sells chia, [but] he throws in, he
introduces weed seeds, chaff, the shriveled seeds. . . . The wrinkled chia seller
[is] an owner of chia, of chia fields, of wrinkled chia. [He is] one who rubs
it between his hands, who cleans it. Separately, he sells the Chontal variety,
[the kind that] comes from Oztoman, the Tlaluica variety, the Itziocan variety.
(Anderson and Dibble, 1963:75)

Other paragraphs in the Codex Florentino also differentiate between
S. hispanica L. and *H. suaveolens* L. Book 10, chapter 28 describes an illness
suffered by the Aztecs and the way they cured it: "The children or adults
suffering from diarrhea are cured when they drink a beverage made of water
boiled with a certain root called *tzipipatli*. It is also good that the woman
who is nursing the baby or the child with this disease drinks this preparation
too. If the adult is sick, he or she should drink the atole made with a certain
seed called chiantzotzotl, mixed up with the cake of some seed called chian"
(Sahagún, 1579:158).

When the nutritional properties of *S. hispanica* L. began to be recognized
in the late twentieth century, the mistake of calling both *S. hispanica* L. and
H. suaveolens L. species "chia" made many people doubt that the species
named "chia" by modern Mexicans was the same as their ancestors had used.
Once again, the books written by the first historians following the Spanish
conquest clear up these doubts. In the Spanish version of book 10, chapter 18 of the Codex Florentino Sahagún describes the color of *S. hispanica* L.
seed when referring to the chia merchants in the Nahua markets: "The one
who sells the seed called *chian*, which is similar to linseed, sells the white
ones, or others painted as marble, or the seeds that did not grow mature due
to frost" (1579:566).

A veined or spotted color is typical of *S. hispanica* L. seed, which is commercially cultivated today in Mexico, Argentina, and Bolivia. This characteristic is not shared by *H. suaveolens* L. seed, which is black. Because of this
coloration one might think that Sahagún was mistaken when in other passages of the Codex Florentino he talks about pure white and pure black chia
seeds. Given the meticulousness of his work, we have to conclude that com-

pletely black seeds were produced by the *S. hispanica* L. ecotype, like those that are harvested today in Guatemala (Coates and Ayerza, 1995).

Cervantes de Salazar also clearly denoted the existence of these two species: "*Chiantzotzotl*, that is like a lentil, is eaten the same way as chia: it provides protection to the blood vessels" (1554:bk. 1, chap. 6). In book 10, chapter 20 of the Spanish version of the Codex Florentino, Sahagún, when discussing the vices and virtues of the Nahua merchants, describes chiantzotzotl in more detail: "The one who sells chiantzotzotl, which is a seed similar to white lentils, owns fields of it" (1579:569). We cannot imagine Sahagún confusing these seeds with *S. hispanica* L. seeds, since they are completely different and also because lentils were distributed throughout the Old World. On the contrary, *H. suaveolens* L. seed is similar in size, color, and thickness to lentil seed.

Today *H. suaveolens* L. is commercially produced in Colima, Mexico, and in El Salvador and is characterized by its dark brown or black color. This color makes one doubt that *H. suaveolens* L. and the plant named chiantzotzotl by the ancient Nahuas could be the same species, because the Spanish conquerors described the seed as being white (Sahagún, 1579). However, plants of *H. suaveolens* L. recently discovered in Colima produce whitish seeds and show some typical characteristics of domestication. This suggests that it was a crop in pre-Hispanic America (Vergara Santana, Lemus Juárez, and Bayardo Parra, 2001) and supports the belief that chiantzotzotl and *H. suaveolens* L. are the same species.

Hernández identifies the chiantzotzotl plant, which is called *chiantzolli* in some paragraphs, with the genus *Hyptis*. He makes it clear that it is not *S. hispanica* L.: "The herb called chiantzolli has leaves like ivy. The stems have four corners and a palm and a half length. The white flowers are delicate, and they are wrapped in some large cells where the white and flattened seed similar to lentils is produced" (Hernández, 1576:258). According to Hernández (1576), chiantzolli seeds as well as chia seeds were used by the Aztecs to prepare a beverage called *chiantzotzoatolli*. This similar use of both seeds could also be a source of the confusion.

A description of a chia (*S. hispanica* L.) plant is also given by Clavijero: "Chia is a little seed of a beautiful plant, its trunk is straight and quadrangular, the branches extend into four parts, opposite to one another with symmetry, and the flowers are turquoise. There are two kinds of chia seed: one black and small, which contains an excellent oil for painting that is extracted from it, the other is white and bigger, from which a refreshing beverage is made. Both were adopted by the Mexicans for these uses and others that we will see later" (1780:54).

Nardo Antonio Reccho copied the manuscripts of the second part of Hernández's work. This copy, written in Latin, was published in 1651 in Rome as *Rerum medicarum Novae Hispaniae thesaurus seu Plantarum animalium mineralium mexicanorum historia* (Treasure of Medical Things of New Spain or History of Mexican Plants, Animals, and Minerals). On page 234 a picture of chiantzolli (or chiantzotzotl) is drawn, and it can be clearly seen that it is *H. suaveolens* L. not *S. hispanica* L. (figure 4.1).

Today, descendants of the ancient Nahuas continue to use the word *chia* to describe *H. suaveolens* L., but, as their ancestors did, they distinguish it from *S. hispanica* L. by calling it *chía gorda* (fat chia). This came about by changing the Nahuatl word *tzotzotl* to the Spanish word *gorda*. This is confirmed by the Mexican naturalist and botanist Maximino Martínez (1994). He uses the word *chia* to refer only to *S. hispanica* L., naming *H. suaveolens* L. chía gorda or *chan*. In Colima this plant is also known as *chía de Colima*.

It is difficult to accept that the Nahua experts who had such a sophisticated botanical classification would have given the same name to *S. hispanica* L. and *H. suaveolens* L. and were not able to see that the two plants are distinctly different species having very different morphological and physiological characteristics, although both belong to the same family. Their seeds are also easily distinguishable.

Although *H. suaveolens* L. and *S. hispanica* L. are both oleaginous (oil-seeds), and this probably is the reason they are both referred to as chia, their oil composition is very different. The first is rich in omega-6 fatty acids, while the second is rich in omega-3 fatty acids (Coates and Ayerza, 1995). When used in paints *S. hispanica* L. provides longevity and sheen, while *H. suaveolens* L. does not. None of the sixteenth-century references that discuss the oil used in pre-Columbian paints talks about chiantzotzotl but rather always uses the word chia or chian (Cervantes de Salazar, 1554; Sahagún, 1579). In book 11, paragraph 130 Sahagún (1579) describes chia oil and its use in paints: "And with this chia the painters apply chia oil. With it they varnish things, make them glossy. With it paintings are beautified" (Anderson and Dibble, 1963:181). Flax or linseed (*Linum ussitatisimum* L.), which has been cultivated since 5000 B.C. in Asia, is also used in paints and varnishes because of its high alpha-linolenic acid content (Sultana, 1996).

De CHIANTZOLLI, seu planta in humore intumescente. Cap. XXVI.

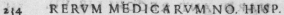

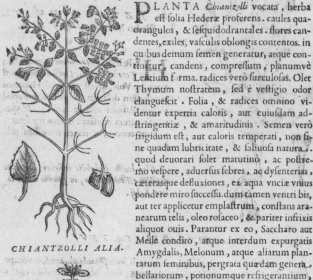

PLANTA *Chiantzolli* vocata, herba est folia Hederæ proferens. caules qua-drangulos, & sesquidodrantales. flores can-dentes, exiles, vasculis oblongis contentos. in quibus demum semen generatur, atque con-tinetur, candens, compressum, planumvè Lentium forma. radices verò surculosas. Olet Thymum nostratem, sed è vestigio odor elanguescit. Folia, & radices omnino vi-dentur expertia caloris, aut cuiusdam ad-stringentiæ, & amaritudinis. Semen verò frigidum est, aut caloris temperati, non si-ne quadam lubricitate, & saliuosa natura. quod deuorari solet matutinò, ac postre-mo vespere, aduersus febres, ac dysenterias, cæterasque defluxiones, ex aqua vnciæ vnius pondere miro successu. dum tamen ventri bis, aut ter applicetur emplastrum, constans ara-nearum telis, oleo rosaceo, & pariter infrixis aliquot ouis. Parantur ex eo, Sacchaeo aut Mellè condito, atque interdum expurgatis Amygdalis, Melonum, atque aliarum plan-tarum seminibus, pergrata quædam genera bellariorum, potionumque refrigerantium, qualis est *Chiantzotzollatolli* vocata, extin-guendis febrium caloribus aptissima, ac bo-num, gratumq; præbent alimentum. quin belli tempore maximi habebatur. quo si sac-cum secum plenum illo ferrent, nihil, quod nutriendo esset commodû, sibi arbitrabantur deesse. Miscebant verò id semen in farinam redactum Maizio torrefacto, atque contrito, vt diutius integrum, & immune à corruptio-ne seruaretur. Cumq; expofcebat occasio, po-tionem parabant, cui interdum succum *Metl* ignem expertum vix Melli nostrati ceden-tem, & paululum Siliquastri solebant admi-scere. Vbique sata hæc planta prouenit, locis præcipuè cultis, irriguis, & aquosis.

CHIANTZOLLI ALIA.

Bellaria·

Potiones nutritiuæ·

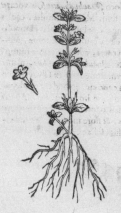

Folia Hederæ similia, longitudinem habent quatuor digitorum, latitudinem verò trium.

Exponimus & Chiantzolli aliam, cuius flos ruber, & folia in anteriori parte la-tiora, vt in Pyrola videre licet.

De·

FIGURE 4.1. Copy of page 234 of Nardo Antonio Reccho's 1651 work *Rerum medicarum Novae Hispaniae thesaurus seu Plantarum animalium mineralium mexicanorum historia* (Treasure of Medical Things of New Spain or History of Mexican Plants, Animals, and Minerals). It shows a drawing of *chiantzolli* or *chiantzotzotl*. (Courtesy of the Biblioteca de la Facultad de Medicina de la Universidad Complutense de Madrid.)

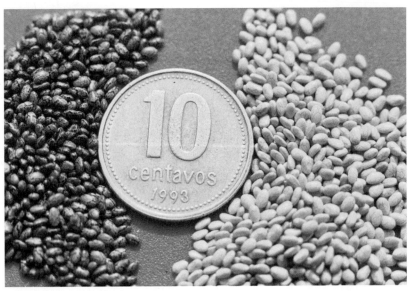

FIGURE 4.2. Chia seeds. The predominant gray and black veined coloration is on the left; the less common white is on the right. (Photo A. Baracatt.)

S. hispanica L. populations that are commercially grown today contain a very low percentage of white seeds, and these come from plants that produce only white seeds. In general, there is little size difference between seed types, with the white seeds being somewhat larger (see figure 4.2). White chia seeds in Mexican markets were reported by Rulfo (1937). This suggests the existence of white and black cultivars during pre-Columbian times, which was noted by Sahagún (1579). The white cultivar was probably lost following the collapse of the Native American nations after the European conquest and is now mixed with the dark seed (Rulfo, 1937; Ayerza and Coates, 1997b).

White seeds that originally came from seed mixtures obtained from the eastern part of Jalisco, Mexico, were propagated in Argentina during the 1990s. These seeds are produced only by plants having white flowers. Differences in protein content and fatty acid composition between dark and white chia seed exist. The dark seeds have a higher protein content, while the white seeds have a higher alpha-linolenic acid content (Ayerza and Coates, 1997b). Although the Aztecs could not chemically determine these characteristics, they could notice that the dark seeds produced higher field yields and better oil behavior when used in paints. This may be the reason that the dark seeds survived and continued to be grown, with the white seeds being lost as a separate crop.

Salvia columbariae B.

In Arizona, Nevada, Utah, and California as well as in Baja California and Sonora the wild species that today is called chia refers to *Salvia columbariae* B. North American Indians use the word *chia* to refer to this species, with the name appearing to be an adaptation of the Nahua word *chian*. This species also has local names such as *dapk* (O'odham) and *hehe yapxot imoxi* (Seri). This chia was one of the most important foods used by Native Americans living in the southwestern United States and northern Mexico, providing them with a nutritious meal and a drink. For Pacific Coast Indians it was a staple, with large quantities of seeds found in grave sites located off the Santa Barbara channel (Gumprecht, 2001). Today seeds from this plant are used as food by natives such as the Coahuila from California and the Tarahumara, Yaqui, Mayo, and Guarijio from Sonora (Munz and Keck, 1959; Prescott-Barrows, 1971; Shreve and Wiggins, 1986).

Amaranthus leucocarpus W.

The name *chía de chapata*, which is used for amaranth today, most likely arose from post-Columbian confusion, as it is difficult to accept that a species with such a low oil content (see table 4.3) could be called chia by the Aztecs, since chia in Nahuatl is used only to describe things related to lipids. *Amaranthus leucocarpus* W., or *A. hypochondriacus* L., as it is sometimes called, is described in the Codex Florentino using Nahua names associated with its nutritive aspects: *uauhqilitl*, meaning edible herb (the leaves were eaten), or *uauhtli*, when specifically referring to the seed (Popper, 1984; Torres, 1985).

The name chía de chapata could have come about because of amaranth's cereal characteristics. In Europe, especially in France and Spain, there is a wheat bread named chapata that is made with double fermentation, giving it a honeycomb structure and a very characteristic flavor. As described in the Codex Florentino, the Nahuas stored chia as flour, then later used it to make a number of different foods. This practice is similar to the one used with wheat and could have led to the name being used to describe a specialized flour used for making breads.

Botanical Description of S. hispanica L.

S. hispanica L. belongs to the Lamiaceae, or mint, family. It is an annual herb, 1–1.5 meters high, having branched quadrangular stems with short white hairs. The leaves are opposite, with a petiole up to 40 millimeters long. They have a few very short white hairs and serrated edges and are 80–100 millimeters long and 40–60 millimeters wide. The flowers are produced in terminal or axillary spikes in groups protected by small wide bracts with long sharp points. The calyx is persistent, tube shaped, bulky, and striated, with white fuzz, having three acute teeth, one of them a little longer and as wide as the other two together. The corolla is tubular and blue in color, with four stamens, two of them larger and sterile. The ovary is discoid and the stigma is bifid. The seeds are present in groups of four. They are oval, measuring 2 by 1.5 millimeters, and are a smooth shiny grayish black color with irregular spots going to a dark red color (Rulfo, 1937; Martínez, 1994).

S. hispanica L. possesses a chromosome number of 2n = 12, the lowest chromosome number in the genus (Estilai, Hashemi, and Truman, 1990; Ramamoorthy and Elliot, 1993). The characteristic stamens and flower shape and color as well as the presence of a nectariferous disc let us assume that chia is allogamous (it transfers pollen from the anther of the flower of one plant to the stigma of the flower of a genetically different plant) and entomophilous (it is pollinated by insects) (Ramamoorthy and Elliot, 1993; Hernández Gómez, 1994). Table 4.4 lists other morphological characteristics noted by Hernández Gómez (1994).

Distribution and Ecology of S. hispanica L.

The Lamiaceae family is composed of 224 genera and approximately 5,600 species from around the world (Dominguez-Vazquez et al., 2002). In Mexico Salvia is the most numerous genus of the Lamiaceae family. The diversity of the genus in the central highlands of Mexico may be one of the highest known for any genus. Botanists estimate that in Mexico there are 275

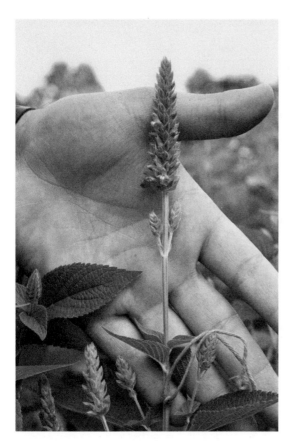

FIGURE 4.3. Chia in the early stages of flowering. (Photo A. Baracatt.)

species, 88 percent of them endemic, with the genus having moved into all possible habitats (Rzedowski, 1978; Ramamoorthy and Elliot, 1993). The major diversity of *Salvia* species is found in the western part of Mexico between 500 and 1,700 meters above sea level, presumably its place of origin (Miranda, 1978; Dominguez-Vazquez et al., 2002).

Historically, *S. hispanica* L. has been cultivated in environments ranging from tropical to subtropical, from frost-free areas to regions where frosts occur every year, and from sea level up to 2,500 meters. Table 4.5 presents characteristics of some locations where chia has been or is still cultivated. The temperature and rainfall values listed are averages over the cropping cycle. Except for Bolivia, Colombia, and Peru these areas regularly experience frosts, and these generally occur in October in Mexico City, in November in Acatic, and in June in El Carril.

TABLE 4.4. Morphological characteristics of *Salvia hispanica* L. from four locations

Source	Seed color	Leaves			Stem color	Petiole color	Flower color	Calyx mature stage
		Shape	Edge	Nerves				
Temalacacingo, Guerrero	black	oval	round or spherical	wrinkled and prominent	green with intense darker stripes	green with slightly darker stripes	light blue	open
Chiepetlán, Guerrero	black or white	oval	round or spherical	wrinkled and prominent	green with intense darker stripes	green with slightly darker stripes	light blue	open
Poblana, Puebla	black	oval	round or spherical	wrinkled	green	green	royal purple	closed
Acatic, Jalisco	black with white spots	lanceolate	serrated	not prominent	green	green	royal purple	closed

Source: Hernández Gómez, 1994.

TABLE 4.5. Characteristics of the sites where chia was or is being cultivated

Country	Place	Latitude	Elevation (m)	Temperature year/season[2] (° C)	Rainfall year/season[2] (mm)	Crop cycle (days)
Argentina	El Carril	25°05′ S	1,170	17.3/16.6	560/390	150
Bolivia	Santa Cruz	17°43′ S	437	24.6/22.8	1,141/566	150
Colombia[1]	La Unión	4°32′ N	920	24/23.8	1,118/341	90
Mexico[1]	Mexico City	19°00′ N	2,259	15.5/16.3	579/470	150
Mexico	Acatic	20°55′ N	1,680	18.5/ —	700/553	150
Peru[1]	Ica	14°05′ S	396	21.1/20.4	3/ 1	150

1. Discontinued.
2. Average for the chia crop season.

Chia Production

At present chia is grown in Argentina, Mexico, and Bolivia. In Argentina and Mexico it is a summer—autumn crop similar to corn, soybeans, and beans (as well as tobacco in Argentina) and competes with them for agricultural land. In Bolivia chia is an autumn—winter crop, sown following the harvest of the other crops, and it competes with winter wheat, winter sunflower, and winter sorghum.

Agronomic Aspects

Chia grows in tropical and subtropical conditions and is not frost tolerant. It develops best on sandy loam soils; however, it can be grown on clay loam soils if it is provided with good drainage. Field observations indicate that chia grows well on soils containing widely varying levels of nutrients. Low nitrogen content, however, appears to be a significant barrier to good seed yield. In general, growers fertilize at a rate of 15–45 kilograms of nitrogen and 37 kilograms of phosphorous per hectare in the Valle de Lerma, Salta, Argentina, and at 68 kilograms of nitrogen per hectare in Acatic, Jalisco, Mexico. More research is needed to establish precise fertilizer requirements.

Chia is sown at a rate of 6–8 kilograms per hectare, with row spacings

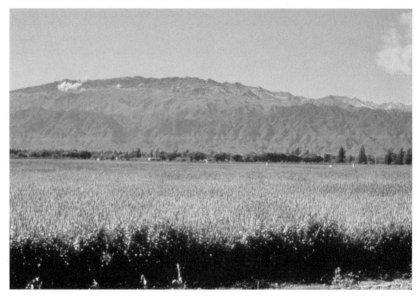

FIGURE 4.4. Field of chia growing in northwestern Argentina. (Photo W. Coates.)

of 0.70 or 0.80 meter in Argentina and Bolivia and 0.75 meter in Mexico. Seedbeds need to be well tilled and free of large soil clods, well drained, and fairly level to help prevent rain from washing away the small seeds. The seed must be planted no more than 10 millimeters deep. Rain can cause soil crusting and inhibit growth. Chia seeds require wet soil to germinate, but once the seedlings are established chia does well with limited water and can grow under a wide range of precipitation. It can be dry-farmed, receiving only 400 millimeters of rainfall as in Valle de Lerma, Salta, or it can be grown with up to 1,100 millimeters of rainfall as in Valle del Cauca, Colombia. In both locations good seed yields have been recorded.

The first forty-five days of growth are critical, because chia grows very slowly and weeds can compete for light, nutrients, and water. As no herbicide has been approved for chia, previous weed control in the field is of utmost importance. Once the stand is established chia can be mechanically weeded until the canopy closes. The broad leaves and erect habit of the plant quickly create a closed canopy, and weeds then become only a minor problem under most conditions. Growers in the Acatic region weed their chia fields manually, with an average of three passes made per growth cycle. In

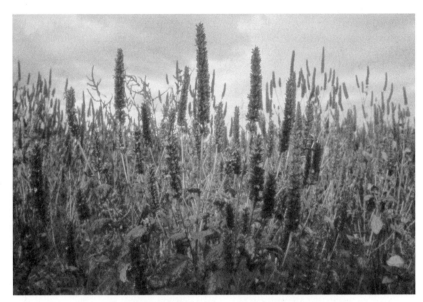

FIGURE 4.5. Chia in the latter stages of flowering. Some heads are ready to harvest, others are not. (Photo W. Coates.)

Argentina and Colombia weeds are mechanically controlled, typically needing two or three passes before the canopy closes, which prevents weeds from growing.

Pests and diseases are not well documented, and more study is needed; however, observations in commercial fields have not shown many problems. The biggest problem in Argentina, Bolivia, and Colombia during the initial period of growth has been ants, and consequently it is necessary to control these insects. Ant attacks have left large spots completely void of chia seedlings.

The genetic material used in Argentina and Bolivia is sufficiently uniform to allow machine harvest. A standard combine can be used; however, some modifications are needed to improve performance. These include providing the reel with sufficient lift so that in taller stands it does not break off inflorescences (seed heads) and cause high losses, and replacing the lower sieve with a 3-millimeter fixed screen (Coates and Ayerza, 1998). The main difficulty with mechanical harvesting is that the central flower head matures and dries out, while numerous inflorescences on side branches remain green. To wait until all seeds are dry means an extended period of time that the early-maturing seeds must remain on the plant. This increases the risk of losses to poor weather conditions (rainfall, winds, etc.) or to other natural causes such as birds. Chia has a large amount of foliage, which dries more quickly in ecosystems that have no rainfall or experience frost during harvest, making harvesting easier.

As chia is sensitive to day length, the growing season depends on the latitude where it is planted. For instance, one chia cultivar sown in La Unión, Valle del Cauca, Colombia, is ready to be harvested in 90 days, while the same one sown in El Carril, Salta, Argentina, needs 150 days (table 4.5). At higher latitudes like Choele-Choel (39°11′ S), Argentina, and Tucson (32°14′ N), Arizona, chia does not produce seeds because the plant is killed by frost before the flowers set (Coates and Ayerza, 1996, 1997, 1998).

Seed and Oil Production

In general, chia has been cultivated in tropical and subtropical latitudes. This was the case for the ancient Nahuas in the Central Valley of Mexico and at present in Los Altos de Jalisco, Mexico, and Valle de Lerma, Argentina, located 2,200, 1,800, and 1,500 meters above sea level, respectively. A higher elevation makes the climate of these regions more temperate than that found at the same latitude but located at sea level (Miller, 1975).

Commercial seed yields generally are 500–600 kilograms per hectare; however, some growers in Salta and Acatic have obtained yields up to 1,260 and 1,000 kilograms per hectare, respectively (Coates and Ayerza, 1998; J. de Rosas, Acatic, Jalisco, Mexico, personal communication, 1993). Experimental plots in Salta yielded 2,500 kilograms per hectare when irrigation and nitrogen fertilizer were applied. Germplasm from Guatemala gave seed yields varying between 340 and 460 kilograms per hectare in Argentina (Coates and Ayerza, 1995). Such variations in yield indicate the need to select germplasm that is adapted to a production zone in order to obtain acceptable commercial yields.

Planting date has influenced production in northwestern Argentina. In Pichanal, Salta (23°17′ S), both biomass and seed yields were significantly higher for plots planted on 17 January than those planted later (table 4.6). However, all three planting dates flowered at the same time. The earlier planting produced the highest yield, probably due to the larger plants that developed because of the longer vegetative growth period. Differences

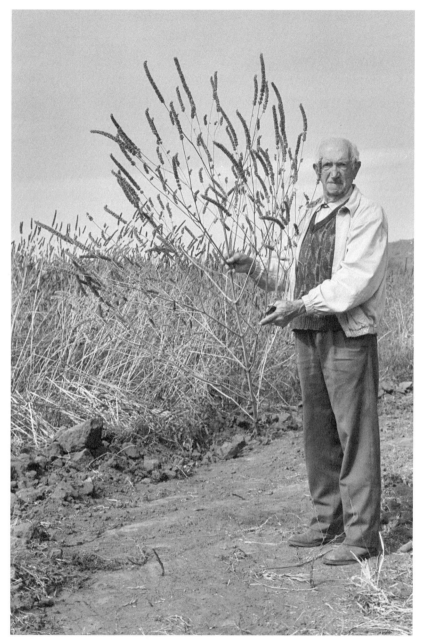

FIGURE 4.6. A single, large, multibranched chia plant held by Emilio Viñuales, father of one of the earliest chia growers in Argentina. (Photo A. Baracatt.)

TABLE 4.6. Effect of planting date on chia productivity at
Pichanal, Salta, Argentina

Planting date	Total growing days	Biomass (kg/ha)	Plants (no./m)	Seed (kg/ha)
17 January 1995	174	3,675[a]	92[a]	862[a]
13 February 1995	147	1,313[b]	47[a]	450[b]
3 March 1995	128	1,000[b]	440[a]	438[b]
cv[1]	0.66	1.29	0.40	
bcd[2]	1,439	852	691	

Source: Coates and Ayerza, 1996.
1. cv: coefficient of variation.
2. bcd: critical difference for mean separation in Bonferroni t-test.

TABLE 4.7. Effect of location on oil content and
fatty acid composition of chia seed in Argentina

Place	Oil	Fatty acids (%)[1]				
		Alpha-linolenic	Linoleic	Oleic	Stearic	Palmitic
Metan	35.6[b1]	63.4[a]	19.8[b]	7.3[c]	3.3[b]	6.2[b]
R. de Lerma	38.6[a]	62.7[b]	20.2[ab]	7.8[b]	3.1[b]	6.3[b]
Sumalao	35.9[b]	62.4[bc]	20.8[a]	7.3[c]	3.1[b]	6.4[b]
Yuto	37.4[ab]	52[c]	20.3[ab]	7.6[bc]	3.1[b]	7.1[a]
Pichanal	32.3[c]	60.7[d]	20.3[ab]	8.2[a]	3.7[a]	6.9[a]

Source: Ayerza, 1995.
1. Within a column, means followed by the same superscript letter are not statistically different at the .05 probability level according to Duncan's New Multiple Range Test.

in biomass weights measured among treatments confirm this theory. The larger biomass volume, however, also meant that more time was needed for the plants to dry so that efficient mechanical harvesting could take place. Drying could be accelerated by applying chemical drying agents, but production costs would increase, and to date no drying agents are approved for use on chia.

Variations in oil content and fatty acid composition of chia are affected by geographical location (table 4.7). This is the case with other oil crops such as soybean, sunflower, and safflower (Talha and Osman, 1975; Carver et al., 1986; Ayerza, 1995; Coates and Ayerza, 1998). Differences between locations presumably arise because of one or more environmental factors. Temperature, light, soil type, and nutrition affect seed oil quantity and quality.

TABLE 4.8. Oil content and fatty acid composition of
commercial chia seed grown in five countries

Country	Oil	Fatty acids (%)				
		Alpha-linolenic	Linoleic	Oleic	Stearic	Palmitic
Argentina[1]	34	63.1	19.5	6.7	3	7
Bolivia[2]	32.7	63.6	18.7	7.1	2.7	7.4
Colombia[3,4]	29.9	57.9	19.2	7.6	3.5	7.5
Mexico[2]	31	61.6	19.6	7.5	3.3	6.7
Peru[2, 4]	32.4	64.2	18.4	6.9	3	7.2

1. Average of five farms.
2. One farm.
3. Average of four farms.
4. Stopped producing chia.

The effect of temperature on oil composition has been shown in other oilseed crops such as soybean, sunflower, and evening primrose (Dutton and
Mounts, 1966; Wilson, Burton, and Brim, 1981; Carver et al., 1986; Fieldsend and Morison, 2000).

A negative correlation between alpha-linolenic acid content in chia seed
formed at the beginning of April and at the end of May and mean temperatures was found (Ayerza, 1995). Similar correlations were also found with
seed harvested in Colombia and Peru (Ayerza, 1996b). High temperatures
probably reduced the formation of alpha-linolenic acid in chia, as has been
reported by Howell and Collins (1957) for other oilseed crops.

Table 4.8 shows the composition of chia oil obtained from commercial fields in Argentina, Bolivia, Colombia, Mexico, and Peru. The fields in
South America all used the same source of genetic material, one location in
Mexico. At the time it was planted the seed had undergone several years of
selection and multiplication in Salta, Argentina. The Mexican data in the
table are for the original seed stock. Clearly, differences exist between the
original seed and later generations, with the differences possibly being due
to environmental factors.

Variations in Chia Life Cycles

Differences in length of life cycles have been found in experimental plantings in Temalacacingo (17°52′ N, 1,499 meters in elevation), Guerrero, Mexico (table 4.9). The differences were attributed to the origin of the samples

TABLE 4.9. Agricultural and phenological characteristics of four lines of
Salvia hispanica L. grown in Temalacacingo, Mexico

Ecotype	Cycle (days)	Height (cm)	Branches (no.)	Heads (no.)	Yield (g/plant)	Seed weight (g/1,000 seeds)
Temalacacingo	102	99.8	9.5	16.6	4	1.1
Tlalapa	112	103.3	9	14.8	2.4	0.8
Chía poblana	115	102.8	10.4	17.1	3.1	1.2
Chía pinta	98	91.2	9.2	15.3	3.9	1.2

Source: Hernández Gómez, 1994.

and suggest that it should be possible to select varieties suitable for other ecosystems.

In one trial the cultivar *chía negra*, which originated in western Guatemala, was compared with the chia now commercially grown in Valle de Lerma, Salta, Argentina. Under conditions typical of Yuto (23°35′ S), Jujuy, Argentina, it needed thirty days more to meet daylight requirements in order for flowering to begin than did commercial chia (Coates and Ayerza, 1995).

In spite of the fact that chia is a short-day species, some plants have set seed during longer days in Arizona and Argentina. It is possible that these could be used to select long-day or neutral-day cultivars, since this is an issue that needs to be addressed if the crop is to be grown in other latitudes.

In recent years crop failure resulting from frost has occurred in the Acatic region of Jalisco (J. de Rosas, Acatic, Jalisco, Mexico, personal communication, 1993) as it did with the Nahuas living in the Central Valley of Mexico. This was described by Sahagún in book 10, chapter 18 in the Spanish version of the Codex Florentino: "It is not possible to extract oil from the seeds called chian, which did not mature because of frost" (1579:566).

Other phenological and agricultural characteristics related to seed production and harvesting practices have been reported (Coates and Ayerza, 1996, 1998). For instance, the genetic material referred to as *chía pinta*, when planted in the Valle del Cauca, Colombia, where the photoperiod is practically the same all year round, allowed four harvests per calendar year. This was not possible when *chía poblana* was sown.

FIVE

Chia and Other Sources of Omega-3 Fatty Acids

In today's market there are four readily available sources of fatty acids, two major and two minor. The former are menhaden (an Atlantic fish of the herring family) oil and flaxseed, while the latter are chia and marine algae. A comparison of the fatty acid profiles of these four sources is provided in table 5.1.

Of these four raw materials, flax (*Linum usitatissimum* L.) and chia (*S. hispanica* L.) are agricultural crops. These two species have the highest concentration of alpha-linolenic acid known (Ayerza, 1995, 1996; Oomah and Kenasehuk, 1995; Coates and Ayerza, 1996, 1998). The other two sources, algae and menhaden oil, are of marine origin. Algae contain DHA, and menhaden oil contains DHA and EPA, both of which are long-chain omega-3 fatty acids. Table 5.2 shows that the terrestrial sources have a much higher omega-3 content than the marine sources. Also, the terrestrial sources contain significantly less saturated fatty acids than do algae and menhaden, another important advantage.

Chia and flax are grown commercially, and all of the field operations are mechanized. Flax is grown in temperate or temperate-cold regions, whereas chia requires tropical or subtropical climates. Fish oil comes almost exclusively from oceanic fishing, while algae, originally wild sea plants, are being artificially grown in saltwater ponds.

TABLE 5.1. Fatty acid composition of chia, flaxseed, menhaden, and marine algae oils

Fatty acids Oil	14:0 Myristic	16:0 Palmitic	16:1[5] Palmitoleic	18:0 Stearic	18:1[6] Oleic	18:2[7] Linoleic	18:3[8] Linolenic	20:4[7] Arachidonic	20:5[8] EPA	22:5[8] DPA	22:6[8] DHA
					% of total fatty acids						
Menhaden[1]	7.96	15.2	10.48	3.78	14.5	2.15	1.49	1.17	13.2	4.92	8.56
Algae[2]	4.2	14.5	27.6	0.8	5.5	2.3	1.7	4.7	27.7	—	—
Chia[3]	—	6.9	—	2.8	6.65	19	63.8	—	—	—	—
Flaxseed[4]	—	5.5	—	1.4	19.5	15	57.5	—	—	—	—

1. United States Department of Agriculture, 1999.
2. Nitsan, Mokady, and Sukenik, 1999.
3. Coates and Ayerza, 1998.
4. Sultana, 1996.
5. Omega-7.
6. Omega-9.
7. Omega-6.
8. Omega-3.

TABLE 5.2. Fatty acid composition of chia, flaxseed, menhaden, and marine algae oils as calculated from the data in table 5.1

Total	SFAs	MUFAs	Omega-6s	Omega-3s
Oil		% of total fatty acids		
Menhaden	26.9	24.9	2.2	29.3
Algae	19.5	33.1	2.9	34.1
Chia	9.7	6.5	19	63.8
Flaxseed	6.9	19.5	15	57.5

Fish and chia both have a long history in the human diet, but flax and marine algae have never been considered important nutritional resources for mankind. Chia was a key component in the diet of many pre-Columbian civilizations in America, including the Maya and Aztecs (Sahagún, 1579; Hernández Gómez, 1994). Fish has been a staple food for innumerable populations living along oceanic coasts. Although the use of fish is declining (Chipello, 1998; Organization for Economic Cooperation and Development, 1998), it is still a basic diet for millions of people.

An important difference among the four sources of omega-3 fatty acids is found when they are used to enrich foods. Chia does not transmit a "fishy flavor," as the other three do. Since the inhabitants of many countries, for instance, the United States, Great Britain, and Argentina, do not eat fishy-tasting products on a regular basis, this is a serious drawback.

Another remarkable difference between chia and the other omega-3 sources is its very low sodium content (see table 5.6). Sodium is strongly related to high blood pressure in humans. Uncontrolled high blood pressure increases the risk of suffering strokes, heart attacks, heart failure, or kidney failure (American Heart Association, 2003b). Recommendations of the American Heart Association indicate that healthy American adults should keep their sodium intake to less than 2,400 milligrams per day, or one teaspoon. Chia seeds contain 1.8, 2.6, 3.5, and 163 times less sodium per 100 grams of an edible portion than do flaxseeds, canned tuna in water, pink salmon, and algae (*Schizochytrium* sp.), respectively (Becker and Kyle, 1998; United States Department of Agriculture, 2003).

Comparing sodium intake between the omega-3 sources when they are consumed by individuals in order to meet omega-3 daily values (1.3 grams per day of omega-3 fatty acids) for a 2,000-calorie diet (Canada [Depart-

TABLE 5.3. Comparison of chia, barley, corn, oats, rice, and wheat

Grain	Energy kcal/100 g	Protein	Lipids	Carbohydrate	Fiber	Ash
		%				
Rice[1]	358	6.50	0.52	79.15	2.8	0.54
Barley[1]	354	12.48	2.30	73.48	17.3	2.29
Oats[1]	389	16.89	6.90	66.27	10.6	1.72
Wheat[1]	339	13.68	2.47	71.13	12.2	1.78
Corn[1]	365	9.42	4.74	74.26	3.30	1.20
Chia[2,3]	550	20.70	30.4	40.29	27.5	4.61

1. United States Department of Agriculture, 2001.
2. Weber et al., 1991.
3. Ayerza and Coates, 2003.

ment of] Health and Welfare, 1990), chia seeds provide 1.8, 237, 78, and 142 times less sodium than do flaxseeds, canned tuna in water, pink salmon, and algae (*Schizochytrium* sp.), respectively. Thus, chia seeds offer a huge advantage over the other sources of omega-3 fatty acids for people suffering from high blood pressure and needing a low sodium diet.

Chemical and Nutritional Aspects of Chia

The composition of chia is compared to the world's five major cereal crops in table 5.3. The protein, lipid, fiber, and energy contents of chia are significantly higher than the other crops. Thus, although chia seed serves mainly as a source of omega-3 fatty acids, it also contains a number of other components that are important for human nutrition.

One aspect of any food source that must be considered is allergies. A study conducted in the United Kingdom (Atkinson, 2003) to determine potential food allergens of chia found no evidence that chia exhibited any allergic response. This was the case even with individuals having peanut and tree nut allergies.

Oil Content and Fatty Acid Composition

Chia seed has an oil content that ranges between 29 and 33 percent (table 5.4). The oil contains the highest percentage of alpha-linolenic acid known (62–64 percent) (Ayerza, 1995).

TABLE 5.4. Protein content, oil content, peroxide index, and fatty acid composition of chia seeds cultivated at nine locations in Argentina, Bolivia, Colombia, and Peru

Site	Country	Protein %	Oil	Peroxide index Milliequivalents of O_2/kg	Palmitic	Stearic	Oleic	Linoleic	Linolenic	Saturated	Polyunsaturated (%)
La Peña	Colombia	20.3[b1]	29.5[d]	3.7[ab]	7.3[c]	3.4[a]	3.4[c]	18[g]	63.2[b]	10.6[ab]	81.2[c]
Jaho	Colombia	19.7[c]	31.1[b]	3[ab]	7.7[a]	3.5[a]	3.5[c]	19.3[c]	57.5[f]	11.1[a]	76.7[c]
Yoshioka	Colombia	18.7[d]	30.2[c]	3.1[ab]	7.6[a]	3.6[a]	10.3[b]	19.1[c]	58.6[c]	11.1[a]	77.6[d]
El Torrente	Colombia	19.8[c]	28.8[e]	3.3[ab]	7.7[a]	3.6[a]	13.3[a]	20.5[b]	54.2[g]	11.2[a]	74.7[f]
La Población	Argentina	20.7[b]	30.4[c]	3.8[a]	6.6[e]	2.9[b]	7.2[c]	20.3[c]	62[c]	9.5[d]	82.3[b]
La Invernada	Argentina	19.6[c]	28.5[e]	2.9[ab]	7.4[b]	2.8[c]	6.8[d]	20.1[d]	62.2[c]	10.6[ab]	82.3[b]
C. del Valle	Argentina	18.8[d]	32.5[a]	3.5[ab]	6.9[d]	2.8[c]	6.9[d]	21.1[a]	61.7[d]	9.7[cd]	82.7[a]
Cerro Prieto	Peru	23.1[a]	32.4[a]	2.7[b]	7.2[c]	3[b]	6.9[d]	18.4[f]	64.2[a]	10[bc]	82.5[ab]
LSD (.05)[2]		0.42	0.39	0.98	0.14	0.17	0.19	0.19	0.27	0.57	0.25
Santa Cruz	Bolivia	—	32.7	—	7.4	2.7	7.1	18.7	63.6	10.1	82.3

Source: Adapted from Ayerza and Coates, 2003.
1. Within a column, means followed by the same superscript letter are not statistically different at the .05 probability level according to Duncan's Multiple Range Test.
2. Least significance difference at .05 level.

Bushway et al. (1984) reported that fractionation of chia seed oil produced neutral lipid, glycolipid, and phospholipid fractions amounting to 97.1, 2, and 0.9 percent of total lipids, respectively. Although the fatty acid profile of the latter two fractions is similar, major differences in composition between these two fractions and the neutral lipid fraction exist. The predominant fatty acids in the glycolipid and phospholipid fractions are palmitic and linoleic, while in the neutral fraction the fatty acid is alpha-linolenic. The ratio of unsaturated to saturated fatty acids is 6.5:1, 1.2:1, and 1.7:1 for the neutral lipid, glycolipid, and phospholipid fractions, respectively. This indicates a higher degree of saturation in the two polar lipids.

Chia seed possesses the highest combined alpha-linolenic and linoleic acid percentage (82.3 percent) of all crops. This is followed by safflower, flaxseed, and sunflower at 75, 72, and 67 percent, respectively. The difference between chia, safflower, and sunflower is even more significant if one considers that they contain minimal amounts of alpha-linolenic acid. Rapeseed and olive oils, like chia oil, are highly unsaturated (67 and 82 percent, respectively), but this arises because of a high oleic (monounsaturated) content. Thus, these two oils have relatively low polyunsaturated fatty acid contents, 27 and 11 percent, respectively (Ting et al., 1990; Ucciani, 1995), compared to chia, which has 82.3 percent.

Protein Content and Amino Acid Composition

Chia seed possesses 19–23 percent protein (table 5.3). This is higher than traditional cereals such as wheat (13.7 percent), corn (9.4 percent), rice (6.5 percent), oats (16.9 percent), and barley (12.5 percent).

Chia seed protein is free of gluten, unlike cereal grains. Gluten causes celiac disease. The Argentina Celiac Association has tested chia and found it to be free of gluten; thus, it has been endorsed for use by celiac patients. A symbol on the label of chia sold in Argentina advises that it is a gluten-free food according to the Argentine food-coding system (Asociación Celíaca Argentina, 2003).

The amino acids found in chia protein are shown in table 5.5. From a percentage standpoint, lysine content is quite high, and methionine plus cystine compares favorably with other oilseeds (Ting et al., 1990). The amino acids in chia have no limiting factors in the adult diet (Ting et al., 1990; Weber et al., 1991). This means that chia can be incorporated into human

TABLE 5.5. Amino acid content of chia seed protein hydrolysate

Amino Acid	Chia (solvent extracted) (g/16 g N)	Chia (press extracted)
Aspartic acid	7.64	7.36
Threonine	3.43	3.23
Serine	4.86	4.43
Glutamic acid	12.4	13.65
Glycine	4.22	4.03
Alanine	4.31	4.41
Valine	5.1	5.32
Cystine	1.47	1.04
Methionine	0.36	0.36
Isoleucine	3.21	3.35
Leucine	5.89	5.99
Tryptophan	—	1.29
Tyrosine	2.75	2.75
Phenylalanine	4.73	4.77
Lysine	4.44	3.6
Histidine	2.57	2.45
Arginine	8.9	8.63
Proline	4.4	3.92
Total	80.64	80.81

Sources: Adapted from Ting et al., 1990; Brown, 2003.

diets and mixed with other grains to produce a balanced protein source. Bushway et al. (1984) demonstrated that chia seed protein can be extracted at neutral pH. This is advantageous, since it has been demonstrated that lysine and cystine can be destroyed at alkaline pH's.

Vitamins and Minerals

Chia seed is a good source of B vitamins (table 5.6). Recent findings show that low blood levels of B vitamins are linked to an increased risk of fatal coronary heart disease and stroke (American Heart Association, 1999; McKinlay, 2000; Taylor-Chinn, 2000). This is because homocysteine, a non-protein-forming amino acid that is not a normal dietary constituent, is elevated when folic acid and B vitamin levels are inadequate (Herzlich et al., 1996; Selhub et al., 1996). Researchers believe that when body cells dump too much homocysteine into the blood, artery linings become irritated, encouraging the formation of plaque deposits that cling to artery walls

TABLE 5.6. Content of vitamins and essential elements
in chia seed and deoiled meal

| Nutrient | Chia | |
	Whole seed (mg/100 g)	Deoiled meal
Macroelements		
Calcium	714[1]	1,180[2]
Potassium	700[1]	1,100[2]
Magnesium	390[2]	500[2]
Phosphorus	1,067[1]	1,170[2]
Microelements		
Aluminum	2[2]	4.3[2]
Boron	—	1.4[2]
Copper	0.2[1]	2.6[2]
Iron	16.4[2]	20.4[2]
Manganese	2.3[1]	6.8[2]
Molybdenum	0.2[1]	—
Sodium	—	2.9[2]
Zinc	3.7[1]	8.5[2]
Vitamins		
Niacin	6.13[1]	11.30[2]
Thiamin	0.18[1]	0.79[2]
Riboflavin	0.04[1]	0.46[2]
Vitamin A	44 IU[3]	—

1. Instituto Nacional de Alimentos, 2003.
2. Brown, 2003.
3. Brown, 1998.

(McBride, 1999). An elevated serum homocysteine concentration is now recognized as an important independent risk factor for cardiovascular disease and stroke (Boushey et al., 1995; Malinow, 1996).

Comparison of the vitamin content of chia with other traditional crops shows that it is higher in niacin than corn, soybeans, rice, and safflower but lower in vitamin A than corn. Thiamin and riboflavin contents are similar to rice and corn but lower than soybeans and safflower.

Chia seeds are an excellent source of calcium, phosphorus, magnesium, potassium, iron, zinc, and copper (table 5.6). Chia seeds contain 13–354 times more calcium, 2–12 times more phosphorus, and 1.6–9 times more potassium per 100 grams of edible portion than wheat, rice, barley, oats, and corn. Chia seed has 6 times more calcium, 11 times more phosphorus, and 4.6 times more potassium per 100 grams of edible portion than does milk (United States Department of Agriculture, 2001; Brown, 2003; Instituto Nacional de Alimentos, 2003).

Iron levels found in chia seeds and deoiled meal (table 5.6) are very high and represent an unusual level for a seed (Bushway, Belya, and Bushway, 1981). Comparing the iron content of chia seed with other traditional products that are known as iron-rich sources shows chia to have 6, 1.8, and 2.4 times more iron per 100 grams of edible portion than spinach, lentils, and beef liver, respectively (United States Department of Agriculture, 2001; Brown, 2003).

Antioxidants

Water and methanol extracts of chia seed meal left following pressing to remove the oil have demonstrated strong antioxidant activity (Taga, Miller, and Pratt, 1984). These antioxidants make chia a very stable source of omega-3 fatty acids and explain why the Aztecs were able to store chia seed and flour for extended periods of time without them becoming rancid.

The most important antioxidants in chia are chlorogenic acid and caffeic acid as well as myricetin, quercetin, and kaempferol flavonols (table 5.7). These compounds are both primary and synergistic antioxidants and contribute in a major way to the strong antioxidant activity of chia (Taga, Miller, and Pratt, 1984; Castro-Martínez, Pratt, and Miller, 1986). Research has shown that quercetin is a powerful antioxidant that can prevent oxidation of lipids, proteins, and DNA and that its antioxidant properties are significantly more effective than nonorthohydroxy flavonol compounds (Makris and Rossiter, 2001). Caffeic acid and chlorogenic acid, both of which are found in chia, have been shown to exhibit strong free radical and superoxide scavenging activity and to inhibit lipid peroxidation. These antioxidant properties are significantly stronger than those of ferulic acid as well as common antioxidants such as vitamin C (ascorbic acid) and vitamin E (alpha-tocopherol) (Kweon, Hwang, and Sung, 2001).

Epidemiological studies indicate that consumption of high levels of flavonol-rich foods and beverages may protect against CHD (Hertog et al., 1993; Hertog, Kromhout, and Aravanis, 1995; Hertog and Hollman, 1996; Cook and Samaman, 1996; Knekt et al., 1996), stroke (Keli et al., 1996), lung

TABLE 5.7. Concentration of antioxidants found in chia seed extracts

Compound	Concentration (molecular weight in g/kg of chia seed)
1. Nonhydrolyzed	
Flavonols	—
Cinnamic acids	
Caffeic acid	6.6×10^{-3}
Chlorogenic acid	7.1×10^{-3}
2. Hydrolyzed	
Flavonols	
Myricetin	3.1×10^{-3}
Quercetin	0.2×10^{-3}
Kaempferol	1.1×10^{-3}
Cinnamic acids	
Caffeic acid	13.5×10^{-3}

Source: Taga, Miller, and Pratt, 1984.

cancer (Knekt et al., 1997), and stomach cancer (García Closas et al., 1999). In particular, flavonoids such as quercetin have been reported to inhibit platelet adhesion to collagen and collagen-induced platelet aggregates and could explain the relationship between these antioxidants and a decreased risk of cardiovascular disease (Pignatelli et al., 2000; Hirovonen et al., 2001).

Lipid oxidation in foods is a problem, particularly with polyunsaturated omega-6 and omega-3 fatty acids. If not controlled, oxidation not only produces off-flavors in food (typically a fishy flavor) but also promotes aging and the degenerative diseases of aging such as cancer, cardiovascular diseases, cataracts, immune system decline, and brain dysfunction (Okuyama, Kobayashi, and Watanabe, 1997). In foods containing antioxidants, oxidation and loss of palatability due to generation of off-flavors are slowed. Synthetic as well as natural antioxidants can be added to foods; however, recent trends have been away from synthetic products because of the suspicion that these compounds may promote carcinogenicity (White and Xing, 1997).

Chia, when used as an omega-3 source, does not require the use of artificial antioxidants such as vitamins. Antioxidant vitamins have been shown to nullify the protector effects of cardiovascular drugs. Recent research found that antioxidants such as vitamin E, vitamin C, and beta-carotene reduce the increase in high-density lipoprotein (HDL) cholesterol levels achieved by the drug simvastatin, a cardiovascular protection compound (Brown et al., 2001).

Since oxidation in chia is minimal to nonexistent, it offers significant potential within the food industry compared to EPA and DHA sources such as marine products as well as other alpha-linolenic acid sources such as flax, since these exhibit rapid decomposition due to an absence of antioxidants.

Dietary Fiber

Dietary fiber has been found to improve the management of diabetes mellitus and aids in the prevention of coronary artery disease and a number of chronic disorders. For these reasons a variety of groups recommend consumption of dietary fiber to be 25 grams per day. A range of 20–35 grams is desirable, with the fiber coming from both soluble and insoluble sources.

The beneficial effects of consuming a high-carbohydrate, high-fiber, low-fat diet on blood glucose levels have been demonstrated (Odea et al., 1989). Soluble fiber increases intestinal transit time, delays gastric emptying, and slows the rate of glucose absorption, thereby reducing cholesterol absorption (Anderson et al., 1984; Marlett et al., 1994). These actions lower postprandial blood glucose and decrease both total and LDL cholesterol concentrations. According to the American Association of Cereal Chemists, "One of the means of directly measuring an immediate physiological effect of dietary fiber and high fiber foods is the attenuation of glucose level in the blood for several hours after ingestion of the food" (2001:120). Comparing the fiber content of chia with traditional cereals, chia seed has 1.6, 2.3, 2.6, 8.3, and 9.8 times more fiber per 100 grams of an edible portion than barley, wheat, oats, corn, and rice, respectively (table 5.3).

Cereal fibers of medium to large particle size appear to have little effect on small intestine absorption (Jenkins et al., 1994). Chia seed contains 5 percent soluble fiber, which appears as clear mucilage when it is placed in water. This remains tightly bound to the seed and has a very large molecular weight, averaging 1.5×10^6 daltons (Lin, Daniel, and Whistler, 1994). The high viscosity of chia mucilage renders it more likely to produce desired metabolic effects than lower viscosity dietary fibers such as guar or beta-glucan (Wood et al., 1989). Hence, chia is useful as a dietary fiber and because of this may possess application in the food industry (Whistler, 1982; International Flora Technologies, 1990; Weber et al., 1991; Lin, Daniel, and Whistler, 1994).

Essential Oils

Chia biomass (the leaves in particular) has an abundance of essential oils. These oils are of interest for their potential flavoring and fragrance values and because the foliage seems to deter whitefly and other insect attacks.

Of the fifty-two components detected in leaf oil obtained from chia cultivated in California, Texas, and Salta, Argentina, the dominant ones were beta-caryophyllene (13.3–35.7 percent), globulol (12.8–23.4 percent), gamma-muurolene (4.4–17.6 percent), beta-pinene (2.5–15.1 percent), alpha-humulene (3–6.1 percent), germacrene-B (1.8–5 percent), and widdrol (1.3–2.4 percent); the lesser ones were beta-bourbonene, linalool, valencene, and tau-cadinol. The dominant components were origin dependent. The dominant component in the South Texas sample was beta-caryophyllene (36 percent), while globulol was the dominant component in the samples obtained from plants grown in Southern California (22 percent) and northwestern Argentina (13 percent) (Ahmed, Ting, and Scora, 1994).

Other Sources of Omega-3 Fatty Acids

Flaxseed

Flaxseed has been used by humans for four thousand years (Schery, 1972). Although attempts have been made to show flaxseed being used as a staple food, it was never used or even considered as a food by any civilization. However, industrial products such as fiber for clothing and oil for lighting were made from the stalks and seeds, respectively, by a number of ancient cultures such as the Greeks, Romans, Egyptians, and Arabs (Cooley, 1899; Gil, 1975; Crawford, 1979; Palagia, 1984; Mayerson, 1997). Flax is mentioned eighty-nine times in the Bible (Moldenke and Moldenke, 1952); however, it is never referred to as a food but rather as a source of fiber for clothing.

Flax has been questioned as a food because it contains a number of factors that interfere with the normal development of humans and animals. The concern about human use of flax is due mainly to the presence of toxic cianoglicosides (limarin), vitamin B_6 antagonist factors (Butler, Bailey, and Kennedy, 1965; Stitt, 1988; Center for Alternative Plant and Animal Products, 1995; Vetter, 2000) and other antinutritional factors, including cyanogenic glycosides, trypsin inhibitors, phytic acid, allergens, and goitrogens (Madhusudhan et al., 1986; Bhatty, 1993; Treviño et al., 2000). All flax varieties contain these antinutritional factors. This includes FP967, a genetically modified variety that has a concentration of cyanogenic compounds (linamarin, linustatin, and neolinustatin) no different from traditional varieties (Canadian Food Inspection Agency, 1998).

The antagonistic factors of the vitamin B group that are found in flaxseeds have been specified as a risk factor for human health. Recent findings show that low blood levels of B vitamins are linked with an increased risk of fatal coronary heart disease and stroke (American Heart Association, 1999). (See the discussion on vitamins earlier in this chapter.) Research on animals has brought to light concerns about the negative influence that flax has on pregnancy and reproductive development. These effects have been attributed to a compound known as diclycoside ecoisolariciresinol (SDG), which through microbial action suppresses the effect of estrogen in mammals. Flax is known to be the richest source of SDG, and therefore special caution is recommended if it is consumed during pregnancy and lactation (Toug, Chen, and Thompson, 1998; Rickard and Thompson, 1998). Both the complex ester form of SDG and the free form of SDG remain stable when flaxseeds are baked in bread (Muir and Westcott, 2000). Thus, commercially prepared bread, muffins, and cookies containing flax carry the warning of being potentially harmful. In order to safely use flax in animal and human diets the seeds should be detoxified. However, the most efficient processes require the use of solvents, and even in the best case the seeds cannot be completely detoxified (Madhusudhan et al., 1986; Mazza and Oomah, 1995).

Human consumption of flax is banned in France and limited in Germany, Switzerland, and Belgium (Le Conseil d'Etat, 1973; Hunter, 1988; Olivier, 1996). The United States Department of Agriculture put a limit on the amount of flaxseed that can be included in human diets. It is recommended that no more than 12 percent be used as a food ingredient (United States Department of Agriculture, 1999). In Argentina the use of flax oil to prepare dietary supplements is authorized by the National Administration of Medicines, Food, and Medical Technology, but the use of flaxseed is not (Administración Nacional de Medicamentos, Alimentos y Tecnología Médica, 2001).

None of the toxic factors in flax have been found in either chia seeds or its oil, nor has chia been shown to be detrimental to animals in feeding trials (Bushway et al., 1984; Ting et al., 1990; Weber et al., 1991; Lin, Daniel, and Whistler, 1994; Ayerza and Coates, 1997a, 1999, 2000, 2001, 2002a, 2002b).

Fish Oil

For many people an important factor limiting the use of fish as a source of omega-3 fatty acids is that fish has been recognized as a potent allergen in both food and occupational allergies. Reactions to fish are among the most commonly encountered food allergies in children and adults (Hebling et al., 1996; James et al., 1997; Hansen et al., 1997; Madsen, 1997). The frequency of fish allergies varies according to geography and exposure. In Sweden about 39 percent of the pediatric population is affected by fish allergies, and in Spain the figure ranges between 18 and 30 percent. A general figure for all European pediatric populations is that fish allergies amount to about 22 percent (Pascual, Esteban, and Crespo, 1992). In France the frequency of food allergies in adults is 15.4 percent and 12.7 percent for fish and shellfish, respectively (Moneret-Vautrin, 2001).

Today only the oil produced from the species known as menhaden has been listed as safe (GRAS, or generally recognized as safe) by the FDA (Becker and Kyle, 1998; Food and Drug Administration, 1999). Fish oils are generally by-products obtained during the preparation of fish meal, and their composition changes according to marine source and degree of hydrogenation brought about during processing (Valenzuela and Uauy, 1999).

Marine oils used in food products are generally partially hydrogenated to ensure stability and prevent rancidity. However, these oils do not constitute good sources of omega-3 fatty acids, since partial hydrogenation significantly reduces EPA and DHA contents to less than 2 percent of total fat content, with the fatty acids being reduced primarily to monenes and dienes (Valenzuela and Uauy, 1999; United States Department of Agriculture, 2003).

In the Netherlands the by-products of herring, which at present is the main species processed for human consumption, are transported to Denmark and Germany to be converted into fish meal, oil, and pet food. The resultant products are of poor quality, as the long transport time allows microbial and enzymatic attacks on the fish tissue to take place (Aidos et al.,

2001). The main effect is increased free fatty acid content and increased oxidative deterioration (Nakano, Sato, and Takaeuchi, 1992; Watanabe et al., 1996). These effects produce undesirable flavors as well as a loss of omega-3 fatty acids. To minimize oxidation antioxidants such as vitamin C are often added. However, recently it has been reported that vitamin C also acts as a pro-oxidant due to its ability to reduce ferric iron to ferrous iron, which can catalyze lipid oxidation (Jacobsen, Timm, and Meyer, 2001; Jacobsen, Nissen, and Meyer, 1999; Thomsen, Jacobsen, and Skibsted, 2000).

Variations in fatty acid composition of fish oil by season, location, species, and so on are well known, with wide ranges in commercially sold fish oils and meal having been reported (Ackman, 1992; Sebedio, 1995; Valenzuela and Uauy, 1999). For example, menhaden oil and cod liver oil have approximately equivalent EPA levels (10 percent), whereas sardine oil contains 20 percent EPA (Alexander et al., 1995). EPA and DHA, the main constituents in fish oils, have different effects on serum lipids, plasma, and platelet fatty acids. As an example, both lower triacylglycerol levels; however, only DHA increases HDL cholesterol (Mori et al., 2000).

Another consideration is that fish oils contain cholesterol because they are animal products. The amount varies by species. For instance, the cholesterol content per 100 grams of sardine oil is 710 milligrams, salmon oil is 485 milligrams, menhaden oil is 521 milligrams, herring oil is 766 milligrams, cod liver oil is 570 milligrams, and trout meat is 58 milligrams (United States Department of Agriculture, 1999). This is important, considering that chia, flax, and algae do not contain cholesterol because they are plant species.

Another concern is that world fish stocks are in decline because of overfishing and pollution of waterways. Serious concerns have been expressed about the potential of sea fish being a world source of omega-3 fatty acids and the ecological effects of industrialized fishing. Recently, Myers and Worm (2003) of Dalhousie University, Halifax, Canada, showed that industrialized fisheries typically reduced fish populations by 80 percent within fifteen years of exploitation. Tuna, swordfish, cod, marlin, and halibut populations have decreased by 90 percent in the last five decades.

Today the high concentration of toxic substances in marine fish is a cause of concern as well. A recent study monitored organic pollutants (sigma-14 PCB, DDT, oxychlordane, and others) in blood of women from six circumpolar countries (Greenland, Canada, Iceland, Norway, Sweden, and Russia). Results showed organic pollutants were, in general, highest among

Inuit (Eskimo) populations, with marine sources being their main food. The Greenland Inuit population traditionally consumes fish and other sea products such as seal and small whales (Hansen, 2000; Helm et al., 2002). A survey conducted on Inuit adults of Nunavik, Quebec, Canada, demonstrated that a significant proportion of reproductive-age women had lead and mercury concentrations that exceeded those that have been associated with subtle neuro-developmental deficits in other populations (Dewailly et al., 2001).

The Food Safety Authority of Ireland conducted a survey to examine dioxin and PCB contamination in fish oils and fish liver oils sold for human consumption in Ireland. It found that ten of the fifteen fish oil capsules sold as nutritional supplements had dioxin levels that exceeded European Union allowable values (Food Safety Authority of Ireland, 2002). These findings are in agreement with a study in Sweden that showed populations consuming high amounts of fish (including salmon and herring) accumulated significantly higher levels of dioxin in their body fat than nonconsumers (Svensson et al., 1991). Additionally, the blood concentration of PCBs in Greenlandic women was 3.7 times the Canadian guideline values for PCBs in the blood of women of reproductive age.

Recently, the FDA advised pregnant women and women who may become pregnant about the hazards of consuming fish containing high levels of methyl mercury. The FDA is advising these women not to eat shark, swordfish, king mackerel, and tilefish. The FDA is also recommending nursing mothers and young children not to eat these fish (Food and Drug Administration, 2001). Additionally, the fifteen-member panel that advises the FDA on food matters issued a recommendation on 25 July 2002 that pregnant women limit their consumption of tuna fish, since eating excessive amounts could expose an unborn baby's developing brain to harmful mercury levels (Neergaard, 2002).

A partial solution to the problems facing fish oils may be aquaculture. However, aquaculture can, because of the feeding methods used, significantly damage ecosystems. Also, the nutritional value of the fish produced depends on what they are fed.

As with mammals and birds, fish do not form omega-3 fatty acids de novo; they need dietary sources in order to meet their nutritional requirements. Although every species of fish has a specific fatty acid requirement, in general and differentially from mammals and birds, most marine fish require polyunsaturated omega-3 fatty acids (EPA and/or DHA), while freshwater fish require omega-3 fatty acids from either alpha-linolenic or EPA/DHA or a mixture of both (Sargent et al., 1999; Weber and Lim, 2002). Some fish, like rainbow trout (*Oncorhynchus* sp.), milkfish (*Chanos chanos*), channel catfish (*Ictalurus punctatus*), and major Indian carps (*Catla catla, Labeo rohita, and Cirrhinus mrigala*), can elongate and desaturate omega-3 fatty acids obtained from lower down the food chain (Hardy, 2002; Lim, Borlongan, and Pascual, 2002; Murthy, 2002; Robinson and Li, 2002). However, other fish, like yellowtail (*Seriola quinqueradiata*), are unable to use alpha-linolenic as an essential fatty acid and require EPA and DHA (Masumoto, 2002), or, like red drum (*Sciaenops ocellatus*) and coregonids (*Coregonus* sp.), they have a very limited ability to elongate and desaturate shorter-chain fatty acids (Dabrowski, Czesny, and Matusiewicz, 2002; Gatlin, 2002). Therefore, in order to produce the typical high EPA and DHA content found in marine fish, a dietary source of omega-3 fatty acids must be supplied through the addition of marine fish oil or meal to the diet. The requirement of feeding 3 kilograms of fish or fish entrails to produce 2 kilograms of fish raises questions as to the sustainability of aquaculture as an omega-3 fatty acid source for humans and animals (Leaf, 2002).

Recently, the issue of contamination has become a subject of concern for aquaculture. During the past twenty years salmon's popularity has been increasing due to its lower price and year-round availability. However, an increasing number of studies have shown that farmed salmon have high levels of contaminants such as PCBs and other organochlorine compounds that have been linked to an increased risk of cancer. One of these studies was performed by Jacobs, Ferrario, and Byrne (2002) of the University of Surrey. They showed that a single portion of farmed salmon can contain more than the safe level of toxic chemicals recommended by the World Health Organization. The authors advise that consuming more than one meal of farmed salmon per month may increase the risk of cancer. Another study that included farmed salmon obtained from countries in northern Europe, Canada, the United States, and Chile was done by Hites et al. (2004). The authors demonstrated that consumption of the most contaminated farmed salmon (obtained from Scotland, the Faroe Islands, and German grocery stores) should be limited to one meal every two months. This assessment was based only on cancer risk and did not consider other health risks associated with exposure to PCBs, toxaphene, dieldrin, and other contaminants found in farmed salmon, since the risk levels of these compounds have not been established. Hites et al. went on to say that "consumption of farmed salmon may result in exposure to a variety of persistent bioaccumulative contaminants with the potential for an elevation in attendant health risk. Although the risk/benefit computation is complicated, consumption of farmed Atlantic salmon may pose risks that detract from the beneficial effects of fish consumption" (2004:226–27).

Algae

Algae have not traditionally been part of human or animal diets, with the exception of fish. The need to use sodium chloride to create an artificial environment in which algae are grown, combined with the use of solvents for oil extraction (Becker and Kyle, 1998; Nitsan, Mokady, and Sukenik, 1999), raises questions about the environmental impact such operations may create in the future.

Available commercial information on the use of marine algae as a source of omega-3 fatty acid in animal feed reports no fish smell or taste in the eggs or meat produced. However, it has not been possible to identify any scientific papers supporting this. An indirect reference about off-flavors in eggs and meat from hens fed algae enriched diets was found in a paper by Abril, Barclay, and Abril (2000). They noted that including up to 1 percent algae in a laying hen diet did not significantly decrease overall egg acceptability in terms of aroma and/or flavor. Although no scientific information could be located, it stands to reason that a high content of algae and the inherent instability of DHA should result in undesirable organoleptic characteristics in eggs and meat produced when feeding hens high amounts of algae.

Some marine algae have shown antioxidant activity that is related to polyphenol content. It has been suggested that polyphenols could prevent oxidative damage to some biological membranes. However, commercial algae shows very low antioxidant capacity. The explanation for this reduced antioxidant activity could be related to the drying (50° C for forty-eight hours) of the algae that is required for commercialization. Jiménez-Escrig et al. (2001) recently reported that processing (drying) and storage decrease the antioxidant capacity of algae due to decreased phenolic activity.

SIX

Animal Products Enriched with Omega-3 Fatty Acids

The Advantage of Chia over Other Sources

Omega-3 Enriched Eggs

U.S. egg consumption (shell and processed) declined from 17.5 to 14.5 kilograms per capita per year between 1970 and 1999 (Food and Agriculture Organization, 2001). A similar trend has been reported in Argentina, with annual per capita consumption dropping from 6.8 kilograms in 1970 to 6 kilograms in 1999 (Food and Agriculture Organization, 2001). This decline also has been reported in numerous other countries where Western diets are consumed. We believe that the decline is most likely attributable to consumer concerns about cholesterol, fat sources, and types of fatty acids and their relationship to CHD (Ayerza and Coates, 2000).

Decreasing the saturated fatty acid content of eggs, especially the palmitic content and the linoleic content, while increasing the omega-3 content can make eggs a healthier food. Clinical investigations have shown that the consumption of omega-3 enriched eggs significantly decreases the risk of CHD (Oh et al., 1991; Ferrier et al., 1992; Sim and Jiang, 1994; Lewis, Schalch, and Scheideler, 1998; Van Elswyk et al., 1998; Van Elswyk et al., 2000; Horrocks and Yeo, 2000).

There are omega-3 enriched eggs on the market today that are obtained by adding flaxseed, chia seed, fish oil and/or meal, or marine algae to the hens' diet. Due to easy and plentiful access to fish oils or meals and flax-seed, numerous trials in which various amounts of these materials have been fed to hens have taken place (Van Elswyk, Sams, and Hargis, 1992; Van Elswyk, Dawson, and Sams, 1995; Marshall, Sams, and Van Elswyk, 1994; Nash, Hamilton, and Hulan, 1995; Nash et al., 1996; Scheideler, Froning, and Cuppett, 1997).

Until 1999 all attempts to modify egg lipidic profiles were done by adding flaxseed, fish derivatives, or marine algae to hen diets. The presence of a fishy flavor in these eggs, however, negatively influenced marketing (Marshall et al., 1994). In addition, a number of these diets decreased egg production due to the presence of various substances in the omega-3 fatty acid sources. Trials that fed chia to laying hens did not produce unusual flavors in eggs (Ayerza and Coates, 1999, 2001, 2002a). Additionally, high levels of omega-3 fatty acids were obtained without bird development or egg production being negatively affected.

The Effect of Flax and Menhaden Oil on Hen Performance

There have been many attempts to use flax as an omega-3 fatty acid source for poultry, though not always successfully. Numerous publications have shown the negative effects that the antinutritional factors in flax have on the development of layers and broilers (Kung and Kummerow, 1950; Homer and Schaible, 1980; Bell, 1989; Lee, Olomu, and Sim, 1991; Ajuyah, Hardin, and Sim, 1993; Bhatty, 1993; Bond, Julian, and Squires, 1997; Novak and Scheideler, 1998; Treviño et al., 2000). None of the toxic factors in flax have been found in chia seeds or oil, nor were toxicity problems evident in birds fed chia (Bushway et al., 1984; Ting et al., 1990; Weber et al., 1991; Lin and Daniel, 1994; Ayerza and Coates, 1999, 2001, 2002a, 2002b; Ayerza, Coates, and Lauria, 2002).

In order to include sufficient levels of flax in a poultry diet to make its positive effects worthwhile, the seeds must be detoxified. The most efficient processes to do this require solvents, and even then the flax is not completely detoxified (Madhusudhan et al., 1986; Mazza and Oomah, 1995). This creates a problem for the poultry industry.

Reproductively active hens have exhibited increased hepatic lipidosis following six months of feeding 3 percent menhaden oil. Hepatic lipidosis, generally referred to as fatty liver — hemorrhagic syndrome, seriously affects bird performance. Van Elswyk et al. (1994) suggest that this comes about because the oil enhances the lipogenic activity of a hen's liver.

Trials with Chia

Throughout the trials with chia negative effects on egg production, egg weight, and hen weight were not found. Key findings of the various trials are summarized in the following paragraphs.

Improvement in Fatty Acid Composition. Feeding laying hens chia increased yolk omega-3 fatty acid content more than 1,600 percent (986 milligrams per egg) and decreased saturated palmitic fatty acid content more than 30 percent. Hens fed chia also produced eggs with an improved omega-6 to omega-3 ratio, going from 17:1 to 1:1, and an improved saturated fat to omega-3 ratio, going from 32:1 to 1.8:1 (Ayerza and Coates, 1999, 2000, 2001; Neely, 1999). These changes greatly improved the nutritional quality of eggs compared with those produced by hens fed a control diet. Eggs produced by hens fed chia yielded lipidic profiles generally in agreement with current recommendations, which are to lower omega-6 to omega-3 ratios from current levels to between 5:1 and 1:1, as made by the Food and Agriculture Organization of the United Nations (1994), the American Heart Association (1991), the British Nutrition Foundation (1999), and Simopoulos (2003).

Egg Flavor. Studies have shown that consumers generally are reluctant to eat eggs that smell or taste of fish (Marshall et al., 1994). Except during extreme hardship and deprivation, food's ability to serve human needs is tied to the sensory values of taste, odor, and texture. A food's failure to meet flavor expectations may often signal a physical health danger associated with spoilage or contamination (Enser, 2000; Wilkes et al., 2000). The absence of atypical organoleptic characteristics in eggs produced by hens fed chia represents a significant advantage for this grain compared to flax and marine products (Ayerza and Coates, 1999, 2001, 2002a). The difference in organoleptic characteristics of eggs produced when hens are fed flax or marine products compared to chia could be due to natural antioxidants in chia (Taga, Miller, and Pratt, 1984; Shukla, Wanasundra, and Shahidi, 1996). Another possibility for the differences could be the interaction between other components in flax and bird physiology (Marshall, Sams, and Van Elswyk, 1994).

Fish liver oils, such as cod liver oil, have higher vitamin A levels than do whole-body fish oils. Increased dietary vitamin A has been shown to reduce vitamin E (an antioxidant) availability in poultry and other animals. Hence, as antioxidant content decreases, the risk of oxidation and off-flavors increases (Tengerdy and Brown, 1977; Abawi and Sullivan, 1989; McGuire, Alexander, and Fritsche, 1997). This probably is the reason for the presence of off-flavors when hens are fed fish products.

Several studies provide solid evidence that including more than 5 percent flaxseed, 1.5 percent fish oil, or 1 percent algae in laying hen diets will result in a significant decrease in egg acceptability in terms of aroma and/or flavor. However, it is possible to include up to 30 percent chia in a hen diet without encountering negative consumer preferences compared to common eggs. Using these values, maximum omega-3 fatty acid inclusion potential in an egg is 175 milligrams for algae, 207 milligrams for fish oil, 214 milligrams for flaxseed, and 986 milligrams for chia without affecting egg organoleptic characteristics (Ayamond and Van Elswyk, 1995; Van Elswyk, Dawson, and Sams, 1995; Abril, Barclay, and Abril, 2000; Ayerza and Coates, 2002a).

Chia versus Other Omega-3 Sources: Comparative Trials. Little has been published comparing chia to other sources of omega-3 fatty acids when used as a feed. Some recent work, both published and unpublished, shows the advantages of feeding chia compared to fish oil or meal and flaxseed for the production of omega-3 enriched eggs. Table 6.1 presents the results of a study by Ayerza and Coates (2001) in which flax and chia were fed to hens.

Considering the similar alpha-linolenic acid contents of flax and chia and the different omega-3 fatty acid incorporation rates in the eggs as shown in table 6.1, it can be seen that chia provided a better conversion ratio than did flax. This difference could be related to the antioxidant compounds in chia that are not in flax and to the digestion process. Numerous dietary factors cause variations in intestinal absorption and tissue deposition of fat and fatty acids in nonruminants. These include the saturated to unsaturated fatty acid ratio (Lessire, Doreau, and Aumaitre, 1996); monounsaturated fatty acid plus polyunsaturated to saturated fatty acid ratio (Chang and Huang, 1998); and total omega-6 to omega-3 fatty acid ratio (Wander et al., 1997). Digestive utilization of fatty acids also varies according to the position at

TABLE 6.1. Cholesterol, total fat, saturated fatty acid, and omega-3 fatty acid content of eggs produced by Shaver white laying hens fed four diets

Chia	Flax	Cholesterol	Total fat	Saturated fat	Omega-3	Alpha-linolenic	DHA
(%)				(mg/100 g)[1]			
0	0	405[a2]	10.75[ab]	3.63[ab]	1.99[c]	0.81[c]	1.18[ab]
9	5	351[a]	9.25[c]	3.02[c]	10.09[b]	8.46[b]	1.64[a]
11.5	2.5	407[a]	9.75[bc]	3.08[c]	12.50[a]	11.43[a]	1.07[b]
14	0	359[a]	9.50[c]	3.19[bc]	12.09[a]	11.12[a]	0.97[b]
	cr[3]	104.8	1.21	5.61	157.1	145.7	53.75

Source: Adapted from Ayerza and Coates, 2001.
1. Per 100 grams of egg without shell.
2. Means within a column lacking a common superscript differ ($p < .05$) according to Duncan's Multiple Range Test.
3. cr: critical range for mean separation.

which the fatty acids are connected to the glycerol molecule, that is, externally or internally (Lessire, Doreau, and Aumaitre, 1996; Innis and Dyer, 1997; Porsgaard and Høy, 2000; Straarup and Høy, 2000).

A master of science thesis submitted by Neely (1999) at Queen's University of Belfast, Northern Ireland, compared eggs produced by hens fed 1.5 percent fish oil and 14 percent chia seed. Chia significantly ($p < .001$) decreased the palmitic fatty acid content of the egg yolks compared to the control and fish oil diets (table 6.2). The capacity of chia to lower egg palmitic fatty acid content was confirmed in a number of other studies as well (Ayerza and Coates, 1999, 2000, 2001).

A study conducted in Pennsylvania found that eggs produced by hens fed alpha-linolenic acid enriched diets made using flaxseed or chia reduced the palmitic and total saturated fatty acid content more than did fish oil (table 6.3). This again points out the effect that omega-3 source has on egg composition.

Fatty acid deposition is strongly influenced by the composition of the oil consumed and by the interaction of oil and energy intake level in animals (Cha and Jones, 1996). Hence, it could be that the different effects seen in the various trials are related to the palmitic content of the oils used as the omega-3 source. The palmitic fatty acid contents of chia and menhaden oil are 5.5 and 15.2 percent, respectively. The capacity of chia to lower the palmitic and saturated fatty acid content compared with fish oil could be related to the difference in palmitic fatty acid content. This is consistent

TABLE 6.2. Fatty acid composition of egg yolk lipids from
hens fed fish oil (1.5%) and chia seed diets (14%)

| Fatty acid | Diet | | | Statistical[2] significance |
	Control	Fish oil	Chia	
16:0	28.49[a]	28.88[a]	24.17[b]	***
16:1	4.31[a]	4.98[b]	4.04[c]	***
18:0	12.78[a]	12.29[a]	12.84[a]	NS
18:1	28.43[a]	29.85[a]	24.51[c]	***
18:2	15.78[a]	12.26[b]	14.22[c]	***
18:3 omega-6	0.20[a]	0.14[b]	0.18[c]	***
18:3 omega-3	2.78[a]	2.60[a]	12.96[b]	***
20:3 omega-6	0.01[a]	0.01[a]	0.19[b]	***
20:4 omega-6	2.88[a]	1.99[b]	1.71[c]	***
20:5 omega-3	0.06[a]	0.26[b]	0.29[c]	***
22:6 omega-3	2.20[a]	4.34[b]	2.91[c]	***
Sigma SFAs	41.27[a1]	41.17[a]	37.01[b]	***
MUFAs	32.74[a]	34.83[b]	28.56[c]	***
Omega-3	5.05[a]	7.21[b]	16.16[c]	***
Omega-6	18.88[a]	14.41[b]	16.32[c]	***
PUFAs	23.93[a]	21.61[b]	32.48[c]	***

Source: Neely, 1999.
1. Means within a row lacking a common superscript are significantly different ($p < .05$) according to the Least Significant Difference (LSD).
2. *** $p < .001$. NS: Not significant.

with trials in which the saturated fatty acid content of eggs produced by hens fed algae or Antarctic sea krill (*Euphasia superba*) showed no difference compared to hens fed control diets, since algae and sea krill have high palmitic contents, as did the control diet (Herber and Van Elswyk, 1996; Grillo et al., 1999).

As discussed in chapter 2, the main dietary factor that increases the risk of CHD is saturated fatty acid content, especially palmitic acid. Hence, chia's ability to lower the saturated fatty acid content in general and the palmitic acid in particular gives it an advantage over fish oil or meal and algae as a source of omega-3 fatty acids. Additionally, available data show that eggs having high enough levels of omega-3 fatty acids to make a practical difference cannot be obtained using flax-, fish-, or algae-based diets without negatively affecting hen performance and/or the flavor, smell, and texture of the eggs.

TABLE 6.3. Cholesterol, total fat, saturated fatty acid, and omega-3 fatty acid content of eggs produced by two lines of hens fed five different omega-3 diets

Diet	Hen line	Fatty acids (%)				
		Palmitic	Saturated	Alpha-Linolenic	DHA	Omega-3
Commercial 1	Brown	22.4	31.1	0.9	1.7	2.8
	White	24.3	33.8	0.9	1.5	2.6
14% flax	Brown	21.5	30.2	4.9	2.5	7.8
	White	22.7	31.1	5.8	2.1	8.1
Fish meal	Brown	23.9	32.6	1.8	3.5	5.6
	White	24.5	33.6	1.9	3.4	5.7
14% chia	Brown	20.8	29.7	7.8	2.5	10.6
	White	21.7	30.4	11.2	2.1	13.5
Purina	Brown	23.1	32.1	1.6	1.2	3
	White	24.6	33	1	1	2.1

Source: Ayerza, Coates, and Slaugh, 1999.

Omega-3 Enriched Poultry Meat

Research conducted to decrease the cholesterol content of poultry meat through genetic selection has brought about minimal decreases and is essentially of no practical significance (Hargis, 1988; Griffin, 1992). However, changes in lipid composition of chicken meat through modification of bird diets has been dramatic. Horrocks and Yeo (2000) reported that women consuming omega-3 fatty acid enriched chicken meat for four weeks lowered their plasma cholesterol and triglyceride levels.

Unfortunately, feeding generally available raw materials to broilers has produced undesirable effects, including retardation in growth and off-flavor in the meat (Kung and Kummerow, 1950; Koeheler and Bearse, 1975; Homer and Schaible, 1980; Adam et al., 1989; Bell, 1989; Lee, Olomu, and Sim, 1991; Van Elswyk, Sams, and Hargis, 1992; Van Elswyk, Dawson, and Sams, 1995; Ajuyah, Hardin, and Sim, 1993; Caston, Squires, and Leeson, 1994; Jiang, McGeachin, and Bailey, 1994; Bond, Julian, and Squires, 1997; Novak and Scheideler, 1998; Treviño et al., 2000).

Because of the success chia had in producing omega-3 fatty acid enriched eggs, a trial with broilers was conducted to determine the effect feeding chia would have on white and dark meat cholesterol and fat contents, fatty acid composition, broiler weight gain, and mortality (Ayerza, Coates, and Lauria, 2002). A summary of the findings follows.

Improvement in Fatty Acid Profile

When chia seeds were added to broiler diets the omega-3 fatty acid content of both the dark and white meat increased dramatically. Adding 10 percent chia to the diet increased the omega-3 fatty acid content up to eightfold in both types of meat, compared to broilers fed the control diet (Ayerza, Coates, and Lauria, 2002). Chia also dramatically affected the palmitic and saturated fatty acid content of both types of broiler meat. The reduction in palmitic acid (up to 20.6 and 12.8 percent for white and dark meat, respectively) and in saturated fatty acids (up to 17.5 and 12 percent for white and dark meat, respectively) indicates a strong health advantage when eating these meats compared to conventionally produced poultry meat.

Not only did chia reduce the saturated fatty acid content of the meat, it also changed its composition: "As the percentage of chia increased, the fatty acid profile improved as evidenced by the change in the relationship of the palmitic and stearic contents. The decrease in SFA content was due primarily to the decrease in palmitic fatty acid. Because stearic acid is considered much less hypercholesterolemic, or not hypercholesterolemic at all, compared to palmitic fatty acid (Bonanome and Grundy, 1988; Nelson, 1992; Katan et al., 1995; Grundy, 1997), addition of chia to the diet was clearly beneficial" (Ayerza, Coates, and Lauria, 2002:833).

Meat from chickens fed fish oil or meal did not exhibit a reduced palmitic or saturated fatty acid content (Miller and Robisch, 1969; Hulan et al., 1988; Hulan et al., 1989; Ratanayake, Ackman, and Hulan, 1989; López-Ferrer et al., 1999). An explanation for the different effects that fish meal or oil and chia had is that palmitic fatty acid deposition remains at a constant proportion of the dietary palmitic content (Enser, 2000). As chia is less saturated and has a lower palmitic fatty acid content than do marine omega-3 sources, deposition is less.

The broiler meat from the birds fed chia had an improved omega-6 to omega-3 ratio compared with meat from the broilers fed the control diet. Adding 10 percent chia to the diet produced ratios of 2.7:1 and 3.4:1 for white and dark meat, respectively, compared to 20:1 and 19:1 for the white and dark meat with the control diet. This brought the ratios more in line with the 1:1 ratio recommended by Canada [Department of] Health and Welfare (1990) and the American Heart Association (1991).

Sensory Evaluation

As was the case with eggs, meat from the broilers fed chia did not exhibit off-flavors. Unacceptable off-flavors have been reported in meat from poultry fed fish oil or fish meal–enriched diets (Hardin, Milligan, and Sidwell, 1964; Fry et al., 1965; Holdas and May, 1966; Miller and Robisch, 1969; Ratanayake, Ackman, and Hulan, 1989; Lopéz-Ferrer et al., 1999) or flaxseed enriched diets (Lopéz-Ferrer et al., 1999; González-Esquerra and Leeson, 2000).

Consumers are generally reluctant to eat poultry products that smell or taste of fish (Marshall, Sams, and Van Elswyk, 1994; Scheideler, Froning, and Cuppett, 1997). The absence of these atypical organoleptic characteristics in the white and dark meat produced by broilers fed chia could represent a significant commercial advantage for this grain compared to flaxseed and marine products and by-products when used as poultry feed.

Poultry Meat versus Other Omega-3 Enriched Sources

Poultry meat from broilers fed chia provides a significant advantage compared to omega-3 enriched eggs. One egg having a similar omega-3 content (660 milligrams per 100 grams of egg) as chicken meat with the skin on contains at least 400 milligrams of cholesterol, versus 53.6 milligrams for the poultry meat. The American Heart Association recommends cholesterol intake not to exceed 200 milligrams per day. This places eggs in a very poor position as an unrestricted source of omega-3 fatty acids compared to poultry meat.

There are additional advantages that can be realized by using chia to produce omega-3 enriched poultry meat:

Poultry meat could provide between 2.7 and 3.5 times the amount of omega-3 PUFAs per edible portion of white and dark meat, respectively, compared to an equal sized portion of canned tuna fish. A serving of 100 grams of white meat from a broiler fed the 10% chia diet would provide approximately 703 mg of omega-3 PUFAs. This compares to an average of 256 mg provided by an equivalent serving of commercial canned tuna fish obtained from supermarkets in Australia, Malaysia, and Thailand (Sinclair et al., 1998). Even when consumed with the skin on, [100 grams of] omega-3 enriched white meat from poultry fed chia has a cholesterol content of 53.67 gm. This is not much different from canned tuna fish (42 mg/100 grams), and is lower than several other types of fish such as canned European anchovy, canned pink salmon, and fresh trout (mixed species) which have 85, 55, and 58 mg of cholesterol/100 grams of an edible portion, respectively (United States Department of Agriculture, 1999).

One edible portion of white meat from a broiler fed the 20% chia diet can meet 46.9% and 63.9% of the daily omega-3 fatty acids recommended, based on 2,700 and 2,000 calorie diets for men and women respectively (Canada [Department of] Health and Welfare, 1990). Thus, daily consumption of two 100 gram portions of omega-3 enriched meat from broilers fed 20% chia, one serving of white and one dark, would match nutritional recommendations for both sexes, and keeps a cholesterol intake less than the 200 mg per day recommended by the American Heart Association (1991). . . .

In conclusion, the most significant findings in this trial were the effects that chia had on palmitic SFA, omega-3 PUFAs, and the omega-6:omega-3 fatty acid ratio of broiler white and dark meats. Enriched omega-3 PUFA poultry meat brought about by feeding chia could be an alternative to fish to help consumers meet health recommendations, without having to change dietary habits (Ayerza, Coates, and Lauria, 2002:834, 835).

Ground Chia versus Whole Chia as a Feed

To date, chia has been added to poultry diets as whole seed. However, ground chia seed may enhance omega-3 fatty acid absorption of birds and the resulting level in the eggs and meat produced. Unpublished research conducted in Argentina as a result of a research and development agreement between Functional Products S.A. and INTA (Argentine National Institute of Agricultural Technology) found that true metabolizable energy of whole and ground chia seed measured using the Sibbald (1975) methodology was 693 and 4,089 kilocalories per kilogram, respectively (Azcona, 2003). This is a significant difference and could affect the utilization and deposition of whole and ground chia seed.

Higher yolk omega-3 fatty acid deposition was reported for eggs from hens fed ground flaxseed compared to whole flaxseed (Aymond and Van Elswyk, 1995). The authors pointed out, however, that in order to avoid potential oxidative processes the ground flaxseed used in experimental diets was stored under refrigeration. These storage conditions would make it difficult and expensive to use ground flaxseed for commercial production. Ground chia has shown no significant oxidative deterioration under extended storage periods. Hence, grinding chia seeds could improve omega-3 deposition in poultry products and would not incur additional storage costs.

Omega-3 Enriched Cow's Milk

In Europe, as in many other Western countries, milk and milk products are major sources of fat in the diet, accounting for 30 percent of total fat and 40 percent of saturated fat intake (Demeyer and Doreau, 1999). Because of this the U.S. dairy industry, as is the case in other Western countries, has seen declining per capita consumption of milk and milk products in recent years. In the United States per capita consumption of fluid milk and cream dropped from 241 pounds in 1985 to 224 pounds in 1996 (United States Department of Agriculture, 1996a, 1998).

Milk enriched with omega-3 fatty acids could bring important health benefits to people of all social classes. Horrocks and Yeo (2000) demonstrated that platelet aggregation in boys who drank milk containing three times the omega-3 content of common milk daily for four weeks was significantly less ($p < .05$) than for boys drinking common milk.

Changing milk composition by changing a lactating cow's diet would seem to be a logical process, following the examples of omega-3 enriched eggs and poultry meat. However, because lipid metabolism in poultry is very different from that in cows, dietary omega-3 incorporation efficiencies cannot be directly compared between them. For example, even if dairy cattle consume relatively large amounts of polyunsaturated fatty acids when eating green pastures, the amount transferred to the milk is small. The reason is that PUFAs are hydrogenated (degraded) by microorganisms in the rumen (Jensen, 1992). Techniques to reduce this process and hence increase omega-3 deposition have been developed. Scott, Cook, and Mills (1971) and Ashes et al. (1992) encapsulated the oil in treated protein mixtures. A simpler process is simply to mix 3–4 percent calcium in the feed.

The main concerns when feeding PUFAs to ruminants are their deleterious effects on dry matter intake, decreased fiber digestibility, and decreased milk fat percentage (Wright et al., 1998). This latter concern affects the price of the milk paid to the farmer, since price is related to fat percentage: more fat, more money; less fat, less money.

Improving Milk Properties

A limited trial in which chia was fed to milk cows was undertaken, and the results were encouraging. The study showed that the milk produced by cows fed chia had 20 percent more omega-3 fatty acids than milk from cows fed the control diet (Ayerza and Coates, 2002b). Linoleic and alpha-linolenic acid contents increased, and the ratio of SFAs to PUFAs improved. The ratio of SFAs to omega-3 was more in line with that recommended by the British Nutrition Foundation (1999) than is found in common milk. Obviously, these changes would make milk more acceptable to health-conscious consumers and could reverse the declining per capita consumption of milk that has occurred in recent years.

Feeding chia to lactating cows produced milk that had almost half the omega-3 fatty acid content of milk sold in stores in Argentina, Uruguay, and Brazil that is obtained by adding fish oil to partly skimmed milk (Parmalat, 1999). Because of the way this milk is produced, however, it does not meet the requirements of the International Dairy Federation as being natural dairy milk (Chambon, 1996). Hence, many consumers are reluctant to purchase it.

While the study did show promising results, the effect of using chia that has been protected from degradation in the rumen at different levels and over extended periods of time must be determined to fully assess the potential chia has in improving the fatty acid profile of dairy milk.

SEVEN

Chia

Markets and Commercialization

For more than four thousand years humans and chia have been connected through agriculture and food. Religious persecution five hundred years ago caused chia to almost disappear, and as a result it lost the prominent position it had in Mesoamerican societies. In the middle 1980s demand for chia was so small that most growers could not sell their production.

For many years chia was sold only in Mexican markets and used as a raw material for making the beverage chía fresca, which was consumed for ethnic and religious reasons. Chia oil was also used in paints by small groups of artisans in Mexico. In 1965 chia seed became available in health food stores in Southern California and Arizona (Hicks, 1966), and at the end of the 1980s Chia Pets had been commercialized in the United States. This increased the demand for chia, and the few growers who cultivated the crop could once again sell their production. However, plantings in Jalisco, Mexico, totaling fewer than 300 hectares per year were sufficient to supply the world market. When the area surpassed 400 hectares, the market became saturated for up to two years. Native populations in Guatemala and Nicaragua also continued to produce chia. In these countries, however, only a few small fields were planted. The seeds were used primarily for domestic consumption in foods and beverages similar to those in Mexico. In some years seeds were also sold in the United States and used for Chia Pets.

Up until the early 1990s information on the negative effects that saturated fats, trans-fatty acids, and an unbalanced omega-6 and omega-3 fatty acid ratio in the diet produced and the advantages consumption of omega-3 fatty acids provided in preventing CHD, cancer, depression, and other diseases was not available. About the same time this information was emerging, results of the chia trials that were conducted as part of the Northwestern Argentina Regional Project were published. This information, which described this species as being a natural source of omega-3 fatty acids, antioxidants, and dietary fiber, increased interest in the crop and led a number of individuals to look at chia from a nutritional point of view. As a result, use of chia as a food began to spread out of Mexico.

Today it is possible to find chia in human and animal foods. Chia seed is sold in supermarkets, ethnic food stores, and health food stores in the United States, mainly in the Southwest. In Southern California a bread enriched with chia seeds has been commercialized and is available in a few locations. Since late 2001 food supplements enriched with chia seeds were available in the European Union, Canada, Russia, and Japan and since mid-2003 in Argentina. Food supplements and energy bars containing chia can also be bought over the Internet.

As animal feed chia is being used as a supplement for horses and to produce omega-3 fatty acid enriched eggs. In Buenos Aires, Argentina, eggs produced by hens fed chia are sold in the French supermarket chain known as Carrefour. A horse supplement named Tri-Omega™ has been commercialized by Vetshare, Inc., of Phoenix, Arizona. Recently, chia was included as the source of omega-3 fatty acid in a formula sold for domestic cats in the United States and dogs in Argentina.

Functional Foods and Nutraceuticals

There are no universally accepted definitions for functional foods or nutraceuticals; however, several government and private organizations have attempted to define functional foods, with nutraceuticals often being included in the definition. The most widely accepted definition is one that describes functional foods as providing a health benefit beyond basic nutrition because of the presence of physiologically active components (International Life Science Institute, 1999).

In general, functional foods and nutraceuticals are used synonymously and sometimes are called designer foods or pharma-foods. Some authors, however, differentiate between functional foods and nutraceuticals; that is, the former is a food and is eaten as such, whereas a nutraceutical is consumed as a dosage. For example, omega-3 enriched poultry meat from birds fed chia would be a functional food, while a capsule of chia oil would be a nutraceutical.

Consumer Interest in and Knowledge of Functional Foods

Interest in slowing the aging process and remaining healthy is increasing in the elderly, primarily due to people living longer in Canada, the United States, the European Union, and Japan. This will continue to increase the demand for functional foods, since the baby boomer generation will be the largest consumer group in the years ahead (Hasler, 2000; Government Services Canada, 2001).

Consumers want to have options when seeking a healthy lifestyle. They search for foods that act as treatments and cures and that prevent deterioration of health (Sheehy and Morrissey, 1998; American Dietetic Association, 1999; Sloan, 1999). In the United States 20 percent of consumers read the nutritional information on labels and buy foods that offer a specific health benefit beyond basic nutrition (Hollingsworth, 2000). A 1997 survey showed that 52 percent of Americans believed that foods can replace drugs and that 33 percent were regularly using foods for treatment of one or more diseases (Sloan, 1999). Recently, the Food Marketing Institute showed that 40 percent of consumers bought specific products with the intention of reducing the risk of suffering from a particular disease (Hasler, 2000).

Research in Germany, France, and the United Kingdom showed that the term *functional foods* is not generally known to consumers. The average consumer considers these products just a healthier alternative. More than three quarters of the people surveyed, however, said that they would buy functional foods for themselves and their families. Of these, more than 55 percent believed that functional foods would improve their health. In the United Kingdom 76 percent of consumers considered foods enriched with PUFAs to be necessary for human health (Young, 1997). In the United States the percentage of consumers that bought at least three products for their positive effects on health increased from 13 to 52 percent between 1998 and 2000 (Hasler, 2000).

As early as 1998 a survey identified research and/or clinical trials as the leading factor bringing about commercial success of functional foods (American Dietetic Association, 1999; Sloan, 1999; Hasler, 2000). Not only are consumers seeking healthy products, but a survey conducted in Canada by the National Institute of Nutrition showed that access to quality information about the benefits specific foods and food ingredients can bring is also extremely important (Government Services Canada, 2001).

The Demand for Functional Foods

Since 1996 consumer demand for functional foods has steadily increased. A study conducted in 2000 revealed that consumers continue to shift their focus on food content from reducing harmful ingredients to incorporating healthful components into their diets (Schmidt, 2000).

In the United States the functional food sector has been growing at a rate of 10–15 percent per year versus 3–5 percent for traditional foods. Today, the market in Canada, the United States, and Japan combined is calculated at $26.5 to $36 billion per year. Worldwide it has been estimated that this market will reach $250 to $500 billion by 2010 (Food Engineering International, 1997; Sloan, 1998; Mah, 2000; Government Services Canada, 2001).

Health and Omega-3 Fatty Acids

In the United States more than half of adult consumers (54 percent) are familiar with the healthy effects that omega-3 fatty acids provide, and 44 percent are seriously considering eating omega-3 fatty acid enriched foods or dietary supplements (Schonfeld, 2002). A survey conducted along the East Coast demonstrated that 89 percent of teenagers knew about the positive relationship between omega-3 fatty acids and good health and that 59 percent knew that consuming them helps to prevent heart attacks (Harel et al., 2001).

In Australia and New Zealand 53 and 48 percent of the people surveyed, respectively, were aware of the relationship between type of food and the risk of suffering heart disease (Worsley and Scott, 2000). In Denmark 59 percent of consumers preferred to buy enriched milk products, with 12 percent of these preferring omega-3 fatty acid enriched products. With regard to bread, 74 percent of consumers preferred to buy enriched brands, and of these, 13 percent wanted bread enriched with omega-3 fatty acids (Poulsen, 1999).

Research conducted in the United Kingdom showed that consumers place the most emphasis on health food claims relating to heart disease, with omega-3 fatty acids being an important aspect. Preventing cancer through nutrition is a topic that interests consumers a great deal, but, interestingly, this is the area over which consumers feel they can exert the least control (Dowden, 2001).

Omega-3 Enriched Products

Omega-3 fatty acid enriched products are becoming more common in the marketplace. Omega-3 enriched eggs and milk are two examples; however, eggs are the only natural food with such characteristics. Although a product known as omega-3 enriched milk is available in Argentina, Brazil, Belgium, Spain, and Uruguay, it is actually a mixture of cow's milk and fish oil. In many countries such a product cannot be sold under the generic name "milk," as it is not considered natural.

Omega-3 enriched eggs have yet to be commercialized worldwide. Country-specific information does show increased consumption. A survey in 1996 estimated worldwide sales at 100 million omega-3 eggs (Sheehy and Morrissey, 1998). In 1998 omega-3 egg sales in Canada (Flax Council of Canada, 2000) and the United States (Brasher, 2000) surpassed 4 and 3 percent, respectively, of total egg sales. In the United States "natural" egg sales (including organic, cage-free, and omega-3) have reached 6 percent of the market share, and this is growing at an annual rate of 10 percent (Andrews, 2000).

In 1999 in Brazil omega-3 enriched eggs accounted for 1.5–3 percent of total egg consumption (Wright, 2000). In Malaysia the main egg producer started by selling 50,000 omega-3 eggs per day in 2000; by the end of the year they had increased their sales to 100,000 eggs per day (KLSE Stock Market, 2001). In 1999 in the Irish Republic 7 percent of the eggs sold by the main producer were omega-3 eggs (C. Preston, 211 Castle Road, Randlestown, Northern Ireland, personal communication, 1999). Another European company, with headquarters in Belgium, currently produces more than 50 million omega-3 eggs per year (P. Surai, 53 Dongola Road, Ayr, KA7 3BN, Scotland, personal communication, 2004). The latest information about table egg markets in Great Britain shows that omega-3 enriched eggs have 1.25 percent of the total egg market value; this percentage is supplied by five different companies with 2, 3, 7, 15, and 73 percent of the market, respectively (Challands, 2003).

Market studies in developed countries show that consumers are interested in purchasing omega-3 enriched eggs (Scheideler, Froning, and Cuppett, 1997; McAllister, 1999) and that they are willing to pay a premium price, up to $2 per dozen (Marshall et al., 1994). Today it is possible to find omega-3 eggs in the European Union that are equivalent in size and color to common eggs but that are 22–110 percent more expensive. In Argentina enriched eggs cost from 17 to 175 percent more than common eggs, while in the United States they are 25–135 percent more expensive (table 7.1).

Milk to which fish oil has been added is sold by Parmalat in Argentina and Uruguay and by Nestlé in Argentina as omega-3 enriched milk. Table 7.2 compares the retail price of omega-3 enriched milk to its common equivalent, with the former costing on average 60 percent more. In the European Union mixtures of milk and fish oil became available in 2001 in Spain and 2002 in Belgium. In Belgium the retail price of the enriched milk averages 77 percent more than common milk.

The Potential Market for Chia

The food industry is characterized by low profit margins, while the pharmaceutical industry is characterized by high profit margins. Consumers are used to paying high prices for prescription drugs and low prices for food. Functional foods provide benefits beyond basic nutrition, as they can prevent disease and promote good health. This allows the food sector and the agricultural sector to become part of the health care industry. Today both pharmaceutical and food companies are involved in functional food and nutraceutical production and commercialization.

Functional foods have the potential to increase production and jobs in the agricultural sector through added sales in domestic and global markets. This offers a number of opportunities for a multitude of stakeholders and includes diversification for growers, value-added growth for manufacturers, and direct health benefits for consumers. Given these potential benefits the development of this market segment is now a priority within the agriculture department of the Government of Canada (Truelsen, 1999; Government Services Canada, 2001; Perrin, 2002).

Functional foods form an expanding market in which omega-3 fatty acid enriched products have become one of the stars. Chia holds a privileged place as a raw material for both functional foods and nutraceuticals due to its special characteristics and the advantages it offers over other available omega-3 sources. The ability of chia to enrich various products with omega-3 fatty acids by feeding it to animals or adding it directly to food (table 7.3) opens a significant future for this crop. It also provides an opportunity for the agroindustrial sector to develop and commercialize products for both the novelty and functional food markets.

Concluding Remarks

Humans have become very dependent upon cereal grains. In ancient times hunter-gatherers ate more than one hundred species of plants and animals in the course of a year. Today humans depend on barely twenty species of plants. This dependence on a few species puts Western civilizations in particular in a very precarious situation if diseases or pests were to threaten any of those species. Additionally, medical and nutritional research has demonstrated the importance of a diversified diet in maintaining human health.

The need to diversify available food types provides an incentive to save valuable ancestral crops from extinction. Cultivating additional species has the potential to diversify agricultural production, improve diets, and decrease illnesses. Additionally, this diversification can avoid overproduction and resulting reduced prices of traditional crops, thereby increasing grower incomes and improving quality of life for producers.

Chia was one of the main components not only of the Aztec diet but of another great pre-Columbian civilization that developed in Mesoamerica,

TABLE 7.1. Omega-3 fatty acid enriched egg prices in Argentina, Belgium, Spain, Italy, the Netherlands, South Africa, the United Kingdom, and the United States, 2001–2004*

Omega-3 egg	Country	Place	Supermarket	Price Omega-3 (US$)	Common[h] (US$)	Difference (%)
Brudy[1]	Argentina	Pilar	Jumbo	1.99[f]	1.19	67
Brudy[1]	Argentina	Olivos	Carrefour	2.29[f]	0.83	175
Brudy[1]	Spain	Madrid	El Corte Ingles I [c]	1.28[f]	0.61	110
Brudy[1]	Spain	Madrid	El Corte Ingles II [c]	1.28[f]	0.60	113
					1.52[b]	23
					1.40[d]	33
Columbus[a1]	United Kingdom	London	Tesco	1.87[f]	1.30	44
Cocorinos[1]	Spain	Barcelona	Caprabo	1.00[f]	0.66	51
Columbus[1]	United Kingdom	London	Sainsbury's I [c]	1.49[f]	1.08	38
Columbus[1]	United Kingdom	London	Sainsbury's II [c]	1.31[f]	0.59	22
Columbus[1]	Belgium	Mons	GB	1.08[f]	0.83	30
Columbus[1]	Belgium	Bastogne	GB	1.08[f]	0.75	44
Columbus[1]	Belgium	Mons	Battard	1.23[f]	0.69	78
Columbus[1]	Belgium	Jemappes	GB	1.19[f]	0.78	53
Columbus[1]	Netherlands	Middelburg	Konmar	1.38[f]	0.87	59
					1.17[i]	18
Columbus[a2]	South Africa	Jeffrey's Bay	Checkers	1.35[f]	1.04	30
Cormillot blanco[1]	Argentina	Buenos Aires	Disco	1.38[f]	0.69	100
Cormillot blanco[2]	Argentina	Buenos Aires	Disco	0.82[f]	0.44	86
Eggland's Best[2]	United States	Mesa	Fry's	2.39[g]	1.49	67
Eggland's Best[2]	United States	Mesa	Bashas'	2.49[g]	1.59	63
Eggland's Best[1]	United States	Pompano Beach	Publix	2.14[g]	1.10	94

Eggland's Best[1]	United States	Tucson	Albertsons	2.98[g]	1.27	135
Eggland's Best[1]	United States	Tucson	Abco I[c]	2.56[g]	1.27	102
Eggland's Best[1]	United States	Tucson	Abco II[c]	2.56[g]	1.27	102
Eggland's Best[1]	United States	Tucson	Safeway	2.56[g]	1.23	108
Eggland's Best[1]	United States	Tucson	Fry's I[c]	2.56[g]	1.48	73
Eggland's Best[1]	United States	Tucson	Fry's II[c]	2.66[g]	1.49	79
Eggland's Best[1]	United States	Tucson	Abco II[c]	2.56[g]	1.27	102
Egg Plus[1]	United States	Tucson	Albertsons	2.34[g]	1.27	84
Equilibrio[1]	Spain	Madrid	El Corte Ingles II[c]	0.88[f]	0.60	47
Flor de Vita[1]	Italy	Trento	Poli Regina	1.45[f]	0.69	110
Gold Circle[2]	United States	Pacific Beach	Ralphs	3.79[g]	2.39	42
Huevo Light blanco[1]	Argentina	Buenos Aires	Carrefour	1.39[f]	0.75	85
Huevo Light blanco[1]	Argentina	Olivos	Carrefour	1.35[f]	0.83	63
Huevo Light blanco[2]	Argentina	Buenos Aires	Carrefour	1.43[g]	1.22	17
Huevo Light color[1]	Argentina	Buenos Aires	Carrefour	1.45[f]	0.95	53
Huevo Light color[1]	Argentina	Olivos	Carrefour	1.49[f]	0.98	52
Omegga[1]	United States	Tucson	Abco I[c]	1.79[g]	1.19	50
Wild Oats Cage Free[a][1]	United States	Tucson	Wild Oats	2.49[g]	1.99	25

*Retail prices (after taxes) in local coin transformed to American dollars on 25 February 2001[1] and 5 January 2004.[2]

a Omega-3 and free range.
b Free range = cage free.
c Different shops of the same chain.
d Organic.
e Vegetarians.
f US$/six eggs.
g US$/twelve eggs.
h Comparable to omega-3 egg in color, size, type, quantity, and production method. When there is more than one brand, the highest price was used.
i Biological (organic).

TABLE 7.2. Omega-3 fatty acid enriched milk prices in
Belgium, Uruguay, and Argentina

Country and city	Supermarket[1]	Product[2]	Price[3] (US$/l)	Difference[4] (%)
Argentina		Fluid Milk		
Buenos Aires	Disco[1]	Nestlé Omega-3	1.09	
		Bell's	0.62	76
		Sancor	0.89	23
		Las 3 Niñas	0.83	31
		Molfino	0.74	47
	Carrefour[1]	Parmalat Plus Ω-3	1.29	
		La Serenísima	0.87	48
		Sancor	0.89	45
		Gandara	0.75	72
	Coto[1]	Parmalat Plus Ω-3	1.29	
		La Armonia	0.71	82
		Coto5	0.61	112
		Parmalat	0.79	63
		Dry milk		
	Carrefour[1]	Nestlé Ω	3.05[7]	
		Nido[5]	2.69[7]	13
		Carrefour[6]	2.29[7]	33
Belgium		Fluid milk		
Brussels	G.B[1]	Stassano omega-3	0.91	
		Stassano	0.55	65
		Joyvalle	0.38	139
	Carrefour[1]	Stassano omega-3	1.09	
Saint Ghislain		Stassano	0.69	58
		Joyvalle	0.74	47
Uruguay		Fluid milk		
La Barra	El Dorado[1]	Parmalat Plus Ω-3	0.74	
		Conaprole entera	0.45	64

1. Data from one shop.
2. Products equivalent in kind of package, volume, and type (half-skim milk).
3. Retail prices by unit, taken on 24 March 2001 (Argentina), 12 February 2002 (Belgium), and 23 February 2003 (Uruguay).
4. Largest difference in omega-3 product price compared to the common product in the same supermarket.
5. Whole.
6. Skim milk.
7. 400 g.

the Mayan. Production and use of chia as a food in this region goes back to very early times. The conquest of America by the Spanish repressed the natives, suppressed their traditions, and destroyed much of the agricultural production system that was in place. Many crops that had a major role in pre-Columbian American diets were banned by the conquerors because of

Food	Chia added to the ration %	Omega-3 content with chia and without chia[3] mg/100 g of edible portion		Daily value per serving[4] %
Eggs[1]				
white	10	742	90	57[a]
brown	10	716	76	55[a]
Poultry meat[1]				
white	10	709	95	55[b]
dark	10	613	112	47[b]
Cow's milk[1]	2	45	34	8.5[c]
Wheat bread[2]	2	427	20	33[d]
Yogurt[2]	2	434	27	82[e]
Hamburger[2]	1	285	82	22[f]
Chicken noodle soup[m]	1	223	20	42[g]
Candy peanut bar	5	1,019	2	39[h]
Granola bar[2n]	10	2,094	60	45[i]
Corn flakes[2]	10	2,045	11	44[j]

1. Animals fed chia diets.
2. Chia added as raw material.
3. United States Department of Agriculture, 2002.
4. % daily values of omega-3 fatty acids are based on a 2,300-calorie diet. See Canada [Department of] Health and Welfare, 1990.

Serving sizes:
a 100 g (two eggs).
b 100 g.
c 244 g (one cup).
d 100 g (four slices).
e 245 g (one cup).
f 100 g (one sandwich).
g 246 g (one cup).
h 50 g (one bar).
I 28 g (one bar).
j 28 g (one cup).
m Canned and condensed.
n Hard, plain.

their close association with religion. These were then replaced by foreign species that were in demand in Europe.

Now, five hundred years later, studies have shown that pre-Columbian diets were superior to present diets. As a result, a number of the components of these diets are being brought back into common use. Chia is an example, and it offers an opportunity to improve human nutrition by providing a natural, plant-based source of omega-3 fatty acids, antioxidants, and dietary fiber. Growing consumer preferences for plant-based foods (except among fans of the Atkins diet), combined with recent studies that have shown farmed salmon to contain dangerously high levels of contaminants, makes chia even more attractive to the public.

The need to balance the essential fatty acid content of the diet by decreasing omega-6 and increasing omega-3 fatty acid consumption, combined with the absence of a safe, renewable, long shelf life omega-3 fatty acid source, positions chia to become one of the world's important crops. Thus, current nutritional understanding provides an excellent opportunity to offer a "new old crop" to the world.

REFERENCES

Abawi, F. G., and W. Sullivan. 1989. Interactions of vitamins A, D₃, E, and K in the diet of broiler chicks. *Poultry Science* 68:1490–98.

Abril, J. R., W. R. Barclay, and P. G. Abril. 2000. Safe use of microalgae (DHA GOLD) in laying hen feed for the production of DHA enriched eggs. In Sim, Nakai, and Guenter, 2000:197–202.

Ackman, R. G. 1992. Fatty acids in fish and shellfish. In Chow, 1992b:169–84.

Adam, O. 1988. Linoleic and linolenic acid intake. In Galli and Simopoulos, 1988:33–41.

Adam, R. L., D. E. Pratt, J. H. Lin, and W. J. Stadelman. 1989. Introduction of omega-3 polyunsaturated fatty acid into eggs. *Poultry Science* 68:166. (SPSS Abstracts.)

Administración Nacional de Medicamentos, Alimentos y Tecnología Médica. 2001. Suplementos dietarios: disposición 1637/2001. 1 August 2003. http://www.sagpya. mecon.ar/0-3/especias/04_Normas/dispANMAT_1637-01.pdf

Agroenlínea. 2001. Bajan 50 percent los precios de maíz, arroz y trigo en 20 años. *Newsletter Semanal* 29:1.

Ahmed, M. H., I. P. Ting, and R. W. Scora. 1994. Leaf oil composition of *Salvia hispanica* L. from three geographical areas. *Journal of Essential Oil Research* 6:223–28.

Aidos, I., A. van der Padt, R. M. Boom, and J. B. Luten. 2001. Upgrading of maatjes herring byproducts: production of crude fish oil. *Journal of Agricultural and Food Chemistry* 49:3697–704.

Ajuyah, A. O., R. T. Hardin, and J. S. Sim. 1993. Effect of dietary full-fat flaxseed with and without antioxidant on the fatty acid composition of major lipid classes of chicken meats. *Poultry Science* 72:125–36.

Al, M. D., A. Houwelingen, A. Badart-Smook, and G. Hornstra. 1995. Some aspects of neonatal essential fatty acid status are altered by linoleic acid supplementation of woman during pregnancy. *American Institute of Nutrition* 125:2822–30.

Aldrich, L., and J. N. Variyam. 2000. Acculturation erodes the diet quality of U.S. Hispanics. *Food Review* 23(1):51–55.

Alexander, D. W., S. O. McGuire, N. A. Cassity, and K. L. Fritsche. 1995. Fish oils lower rat plasma and hepatic, but not immune cell alpha-tocopherol concentration. *Journal of Nutrition* 125:2640–49.

Alvarez, C. 1995. Remedio para el colésterol. *Mercado* (Buenos Aires, Argentina) May:1.

American Association of Cereal Chemists. 2001. The definition of dietary fiber. *Cereal Foods World* 46(3):112–26.

American Dietetic Association. 1999. Functional foods: position of ADA. *Journal of the American Dietetic Association* 99:1278–85.

American Heart Association. 1988. Dietary guidelines for healthy American adults: a statement for physicians and health professionals by the Nutrition Committee, American Heart Association. *Arteriosclerosis* 8:218A–21A.

———. 1990. The cholesterol facts. American Heart Association and the National Heart, Lung, and Blood Institute, special report. *Circulation* 81(5):1721–33.

———. 1991. Report of the expert panel on population strategies for blood cholesterol reduction. National Cholesterol Education Program, National Heart, Lung, and Blood Institute, and National Institutes of Health. *Circulation* 83(6):2156–232.

———. 1999. Homocysteine, folic acid and cardiovascular disease. 11 November. http://www.americanheart.org/Heart_and_Stroke_A_Z_Guide/homocys.html

———. 2001. Summary of the scientific conference on dietary fatty acids and cardiovascular health. *Circulation* 103:1034–42.

———. 2003a. *Heart disease and stroke statistics: 2003 update*. Dallas: American Heart Association.

———. 2003b. Sodium recommendations. 31 July. http://www.americanheart.org/presenter.jhtml?identifier=538

American Journal of Pharmacy. 1885. Materia medica of the new Mexican pharmacopoeia, part 1. *American Journal of Pharmacy* 57(10):5–7.

Anderson, A. J. O., and C. E. Dibble, eds. and trans. 1963. *Florentine codex. General history of the things of New Spain* by Fray B. de Sahagún. Santa Fe, N.M., and Salt Lake City: School of American Research and University of Utah.

Anderson, J. W., L. Story, B. Sieling, W. J. Chen, M. S. Perto, and J. Story. 1984.

Hypocholesterolemic effects of oat-bran or bean intake for hypercholesterolemic men. *American Journal of Clinical Nutrition* 40:1146–55.

Andrade, A. D., A. F. Rubira, M. Matsushita, and N. E. Souza. 1995. Omega-3 fatty acids in freshwater fish from South Brazil. *Journal of the American Oil Chemists' Society* 72(10):1207–10.

Andrews, A. 2000. Market watch: specialty eggs show significant growth. *Retailer Newsletter of the American Egg Board* 2:1. 26 January. http://www.aeb.org/retail/retail_newsletter/spring00/spring-2000.htm

Antunez de Mayolo, S. E. 1981. *La nutrición en el antiguo Perú*. Lima: Banco Central de Reserva del Perú, Oficina Numismática.

Armando, A. B., and G. A. Fantoni. 1997. Dioses y códices prehispánicos en la obra de Xul Solar. *Ciencia Hoy* 7(37):1–7.

Aro, A., J. Van Amelsvoort, W. Becker, M. A. van Erp-Baart, A. Kaftos, T. Leth, and G. van Poppel. 1998. Trans-fatty acids in dietary fats and oils from 14 European countries: the TRANSFAIR study. *Journal of Food Composition and Analysis* 11:137–49.

Ascherio, A., and W. C. Willett. 1996. New directions in dietary studies of coronary heart disease. *Journal of Nutrition* 125:647S–55S.

Ashes, J. R., P. S. V. Welch, S. K. Gulati, T. W. Scott, and G. H. Brown. 1992. Manipulation of the fatty acid composition of milk by feeding protected canola seeds. *Journal of Dairy Science* 75:1090–96.

Asociación Celíaca Argentina. 2003. Alimentos Ancestrales—Functional Products SA: productos aptos analizados por método Elisa. Buenos Aires, Argentina, 4 pp.

Atkinson, H. 2003. Studies to assess the allergenic potential of chia (*Salvia hispanica*). BIBRA Report 4095/4194. Carshalton, Surrey, U.K.: BIBRA International Ltd.

Aveldaño, M. I. 1992. Long and very long polyunsaturated fatty acids of retina and spermatozoa: the whole complement of polyenoic fatty acids series. In *Neurobiology of essential fatty acids*, ed. N. G. Bazan, M. G. Murphy, and G. Toffano, 231–42. New York: Plenum Press.

Ayamond, W. M., and M. E. Van Elswyk. 1995. Yolk thiobarbituric acid reactive substances and n-3 fatty acids in response to whole and ground flaxseed. *Poultry Science* 74:1388–94.

Ayerza, R. (h). 1995. Oil content and fatty acid composition of chia (*Salvia hispanica* L.) from five northwestern locations in Argentina. *Journal of the American Oil Chemists' Society* 72:1079–81.

———. (h). 1996a. New industrial crops in South America. In *Proceedings of the third international conference on new industrial crops and products, and the ninth international conference on jojoba and its uses*, ed. L. H. Princen and C. Rossi, 187–91. Peoria, Ill.: American Oil Chemists' Society.

———. (h). 1996b. Fatty acid composition, protein and oil content of chia (*Salvia hispanica* L.) grown in Colombia and Argentina. In *Abstracts of the third European symposium on industrial crops and products*, 1. Reims, France.

Ayerza, R. (h), and W. Coates. 1996. New industrial crops: Northwestern Argentina Regional Project. In *Progress in new crops*, ed. J. J. Janick, 46–51. Alexandria, Va.: ASHS Press.

———. 1997a. An omega-3 fatty acid enriched chia diet: its influence on egg fatty acid composition, cholesterol and oil content. In *Abstracts of an international conference of the Association for the Advancement of Industrial Crops*, 51. Saltillo, Mexico.

———. 1997b. Selection and development of chia cultivars: initial results. In *Abstracts of an international conference of the Association for the Advancement of Industrial Crops*, 50. Saltillo, Mexico.

———. 1999. An omega-3 fatty acid enriched chia diet: its influence on egg fatty acid composition, cholesterol and oil content. *Canadian Journal of Animal Science* 79:53–58.

———. 2000. Dietary levels of chia: influence on yolk cholesterol, lipid content and fatty acid composition for two strains of hens. *Poultry Science* 78:724–39.

———. 2001. The omega-3 enriched eggs: the influence of dietary linolenic acid source combination on egg production and composition. *Canadian Journal of Animal Science* 81:355–62.

———. 2002a. Dietary levels of chia: influence on hen weight, egg production, and egg sensory quality. *British Poultry Science* 43(2):283–90.

———. 2002b. Influence of chia on total fat, cholesterol, and fatty acid profile of Holstein cow's milk. In *Abstracts of the annual meeting of the Association for the Advancement of Industrial Crops*, 8. Saskatoon, Saskatchewan, Canada.

———. 2003. Protein and oil content, peroxide index and fatty acid composition of chia (*Salvia hispanica* L.) grown in six tropical and sub-tropical ecosystems of South America. *Tropical Science* (in press).

Ayerza, R. (h), W. Coates, and M. Lauria. 2002. Chia as an omega-3 fatty acid source for broilers: influence on fatty acid composition, cholesterol and fat content of white and dark meat, on growth performance and on meat flavor. *Poultry Science* 81:826–37.

Ayerza, R., W. Coates, and B. Slaugh. 1999. Comparison of chia with other omega-3 sources for egg production. Eggland's Best, King of Prussia, Pa.

Azcona, J. 2003. Composición de lino, colza y chía. Convenio Functional Products — INTA. EERA-INTA Pergamino, Pergamino, Argentina, 1 p.

Balick, M. J., and P. A. Cox. 1997. *Plants, people, and culture: the science of ethnobotany*. New York: Scientific American Library.

Bang, H. O., and J. Dyerberg. 1972. Plasma lipids and lipoproteins in Greenland west coast Eskimos. *Acta Medica Scandinavica* 192:85–94.

Bang, H. O., J. Dyerberg, and N. A. Hjorne. 1976. The composition of food consumed by Greenland Eskimos. *Acta Medica Scandinavica* 200:69–73.

Bang, H. O., J. Dyerberg, and H. M. Sinclair. 1980. The composition of the Eskimo food in northwestern Greenland. *American Journal of Clinical Nutrition* 33:2657–61.

Baughman, W. F., and G. S. Jamieson. 1929. Chia seed oil. *Oil and Fat Industries* 6(9):15–17.

Beale, C. L. 2001. A century of population growth and change. *Food Review* 23(1):16–22.

Beaumont, P. de la P. C. 1792. *Crónica de Mechoacán.* 1932 ed., 3 vols. Mexico City: Archivo General de la Nación, Talleres Gráficos de la Nación.

Becker, C. C., and D. J. Kyle. 1998. Developing functional foods containing algal docosahexaenoic acid. *Food Technology* 52(7):68–71.

Bell, B. 1996. Australian linola waits for market demand to grow. *Lipid Technology Newsletter* 2(3):48.

Bell, J. M. 1989. Nutritional characteristics and protein uses of oilseed meals. In Robbelen, Downey, and Ashri, 1989:192–207.

Benavente, Toribio. 1541. Historia de los indios de la Nueva España. In *Documentos para historia de México*, ed. J. G. Icazabalceta, 1858:1–13. Mexico City: Librería de J. M. Andrade.

Benson, E. P. 1977. *The Maya world.* New York: Thomas Y. Crowell.

Berger, K. 1996. The palm oil—soybean oil and the nutritional facts. *Lipids Technology Newsletter* 2(2):36–39.

Berger, K. G. 1989. Problems and opportunities in market development of oils. In *Fats for the Future*, ed. R. C. Cambie, 218–32. Research Triangle Park, N.C.: International Union Pure and Applied Chemistry.

Berkow, R., and A. J. Fletcher. 1992. *The Merck manual of diagnosis and therapy.* Rahway, N.J.: Merck Research Laboratories.

Berry, E. M., and J. Hirsch. 1986. Does dietary linolenic acid influence blood pressure? *American Journal of Clinical Nutrition* 44:336–40.

Bhatty, R. S. 1993. Further compositional analyses of flax: mucilage, trypsin inhibitors and hydrocyanic acid. *Journal of the American Oil Chemists' Society* 70(9):899–904.

Billeaud, C., D. Bouglé, P. Sarda, N. Combe, S. Mazette, F. Babin, B. Entressangles, B. Descomps, A. Nouvelot, and F. Mendy. 1997. Effects of preterm infant formula supplementation with alpha-linolenic acid with a linoleate/alpha-linolenate ratio of 6:1: a multicentric study. *European Journal of Clinical Nutrition* 51:520–26.

Bjerve, K. S., O. L. Brekke, K. J. Fougner, and K. Midthjell. 1988. Omega-3 and omega-6 fatty acids in serum lipids and their relationship to human disease. In Galli and Simopoulos, 1988:241–51.

Bjerve, K. S., I. L. Mostad, and L. Thorensen. 1987. Alpha-linolenic acid deficiency in patients on long-term gastric-tube feeding: estimation of linolenic acid and long-chain unsaturated n-3 fatty acid requirement in man. *American Journal of Clinical Nutrition* (45):66–77.

Bohnet, M. 2001. Status of rural development within German development co-operation. *Agriculture + Rural Development* 8(2):3–5.

Bonanome, A., and S. M. Grundy. 1988. Effect of dietary stearic acid on plasma cholesterol and lipoprotein levels. *New England Journal of Medicine* 318:1244–48.

Bond, J. M., R. J. Julian, and E. J. Squires. 1997. Effect of dietary flaxseed on broiler growth, erythrocyte deformability and fatty acid composition of erythrocyte membranes. *Canadian Journal of Animal Science* 77:279–86.

Bonfil Batalla, G. 1987. *El universo del amate*. Mexico City: Museo Nacional de Culturas Populares, García Valades Editores.

Bont, J. A. M., ed. 1990. *Biotechnology and fatty acids: new perspectives for agricultural production*. Wageningen, The Netherlands: Pudoc.

Borkman, M., L. H. Storlien, D. A. Pan, A. B. Jenkins, D. J. Chisholm, and L. V. Campbell. 1993. The relation between insulin sensitivity and the fatty acid composition of skeletal-muscle phospholipids. *New England Journal of Medicine* 323:238–44.

Boushey, C. J., S. Beresford, G. Omenn, and A. Motulsky. 1995. A quantitative assessment of plasma homocysteine as a risk factor for vascular disease. Probable benefits of increasing folate intakes. *Journal of the American Medical Association* 274:1049–57.

Brasher, P. 2000. Eggs are making a comeback nationwide. *Staten Island Advance*. 30 August. http://www.silive.com/food/advance/0419eggs19.html

Brenna, J. T. 2002. Efficiency of conversion of alpha-linolenic acid to long-chain n-3 fatty acids in man. *Current Opinion in Clinical Nutrition and Metabolic Care* 5:127–32.

British Nutrition Foundation. 1992. *Unsaturated fatty acids: nutritional and physiological significance*. Task Force Report. London: Chapman and Hall.

———. 1999. N-3 fatty acids and health. Briefing Paper, London.

Brown, B. G., X. Q. Zhao, A. Chait, L. D. Fisher, M. C. Cheung, J. S. Morse, A. A. Dowdy, E. K. Marino, E. L. Bolson, P. Alaupovic, J. A. Frohlich, and J. J. Albers. 2001. Simvastatin and niacin, antioxidant vitamins, or the combination for the prevention of coronary disease. *New England Journal of Medicine* 345(22):1583–92.

Brown, J. 1998. Chia seed data. International Flora Technologies, Inc., Gilbert, Ariz., 1 p.

———. 2003. Chia seed and meal data. International Flora Technologies, Inc., Gilbert, Ariz., 1 p.

Brown, M., and I. Golding. 1992. *The future of agriculture: developing country implica-*

tions. Paris: Development Center of the Organization for Economic Cooperation and Development.

Bruckner, G. 1992. Biological effects of polyunsaturated fatty acids. In Chow, 1992b:735–52.

Budowski, P. 1988. Omega-3 fatty acids in health and disease. *World Review of Nutrition Diet* 57:214–74.

Bushway, A. A., P. R. Belya, and R. J. Bushway. 1981. Chia seed as a source of oil, polysaccharide, and protein. *Journal of Food Science* 46:1349–56.

Bushway, A. A., A. M. Wilson, L. Houston, and R. J. Bushway. 1984. Selected properties of the lipid and protein fractions from chia seed. *Journal of Food Science* 49:555–57.

Butler, G. W., R. W. Bailey, and L. D. Kennedy. 1965. Studies on the glucosidase linamarase. *Phytochemistry* 4(3):369–81.

Bye, R. 1993. The role of humans in the diversification of plants in Mexico. In Ramamoorthy et al., 1993:707–32.

Canada [Department of] Health and Welfare. 1990. *Nutrition recommendations*. Ottawa: Canadian Government Publishing Center.

Canadian Food Inspection Agency. 1998. Decision document 98-24: determination of the safety of the Crop Development Center's "CDC Triffied," a flax (*Linum usitatissimum* L.) variety tolerant to soil residues of triasulfuron and metsulfuron-methyl. Plant Health and Production Division, Plant Biosafety Office. 23 October 2001. http://www.inspection.gc.ca/english/plaveg/pbo/dd9824c.shtml

Cancian, F. 1971. *Economics and prestige in a Maya community: the religious cargo system in Zinacantan*. Stanford, Calif.: Stanford University Press.

Cantwell, M. M. 2000. Assessment of individual fatty acid intake. *Proceedings of the Nutrition Society* 59:187–91.

Carver, B. F., J. W. Burton, T. E. Carter, and R. F. Wilson. 1986. Response to environmental variation of soybean lines selected for altered unsaturated fatty acid composition. *Crop Science* 26(6):1176–80.

Caston, L. J., E. J. Squires, and S. Leeson. 1994. Hen performance, egg quality, and the sensory evaluation of eggs from SCWL hens fed dietary flax. *Canadian Journal of Animal Science* 74:347–53.

Castro-Martínez, R., D. E. Pratt, and E. E. Miller. 1986. Natural antioxidants of chia seeds. In *Proceedings of the world conference on emerging technologies in the fats and oils industry*, ed. American Oil Chemists' Society, 392–96. Champaign, Ill.: American Oil Chemists' Society Press.

Center for Alternative Plant and Animal Products. 1995. Flaxseed oil contains lignans which could prevent blood clot formation and aid in brain development. *Bio Options* 7(1):7.

Cervantes de Salazar, F. 1554. *Crónica de la Nueva España*. Ed. Manuel Megallón,

1971. Madrid: Ediciones Atlas. Versión digital de la biblioteca virtual Miguel de Cervantes, Universidad de Alicante, Alicante, Spain. http://www.cervantes virtual.com/servlet/SirveObras/89147396432367251854457/p0000001.htm#8

Cha, M. C., and P. J. H. Jones. 1996. Tissue fatty acid deposition is influenced by an interaction of dietary oil source and energy intake level in rats. *Journal of Nutritional Biochemistry* 7:650–58.

Challands, P. 2003. From Columbus® egg to Columbus® food: strategies for consumer-marketing. Presented at the Second International Congress on the Columbus Concept, Athens.

Chambon, M. 1996. Milk fat. In Karleskind and Wolff, 1996:277–85.

Chang, N. W., and P. C. Huang. 1998. Effects of the ratio of polyunsaturated and monounsaturated fatty acid on rat plasma and liver lipid concentration. *Lipids* 33:481–87.

Chavali, S. R., and R. A. Forse. 1994. The role of omega-3 polyunsaturated fatty acids on immune responses during infection and inflammation. In Forse, 1994:179–85.

Chipello, C. J. 1998. Fishing industry fades as does a way of life in Newfoundland ports. *Wall Street Journal* 131(97):1.

Cho, S. Y., K. Mayashita, T. Miyazawa, K. Fujimoto, and T. Kaneda. 1987. Autoxidation of ethyl eicosapentaenoate and docosahexaenoate. *Journal of the American Oil Chemists' Society* 64:876–79.

Choudhury, N., L. Tan, and A. S. Truswell. 1995. Comparison of palmolein and olive oil: effects on plasma lipids and vitamin E in young adults. *American Journal of Clinical Nutrition* 61:1043–51.

Chow, C. K. 1992a. Biological effects of oxidized fatty acids. In Chow, 1992b:689–706.

———, ed. 1992b. *Fatty acids in food and their health implications*. New York: Marcel Dekker.

Christensen, A. F. 1996. History, myth, and migration in Mesoamerica. Presented at the annual meeting of the American Society for Ethnohistory, 7 November, Portland, Ore.

Ciudad Real, A. de. 1585. *Tratado curioso y docto de las grandezas de la Nueva España: relación breve y verdadera de algunas cosas de las muchas que sucedieron al padre Fray Alonso Ponce en las provincias de la Nueva España, siendo comisario general de aquellas partes*. Ed. V. M. Castillo Ferreras and J. García Quintana, 1976. Mexico City: Instituto de Investigaciones Históricas, Universidad Nacional Autónoma de México.

Clavijero, F. J. 1780. *Storia antica del Messico avata da migliori storici spagnoli e da'manos critti, e dalla pitture antiche degli' indiani divisa in dieci libri, e corredata di corte geografiche, e di varce figure e dissertazioni sulla terra, sugli animali e sugli abitatori del Messino*. Bologna, Italy: Gregorio Biasini.

Coates, W., and R. Ayerza (h). 1995. *New crops for the Río Bermejo basin: phase II—final report*. Bioresources Research Facility, Office of Arid Lands Studies, University of Arizona, Tucson, 29 pp.

———. 1996. Production potential of chia in northwestern Argentina. *Industrial Crops and Products* 5:229–33.

———. 1997. New crop trials in the Patagonian region of Argentina. In *Abstracts of an international conference of the Association for the Advancement of Industrial Crops*, 23. Saltillo, Mexico.

———. 1998. Commercial production of chia in northwestern Argentina. *Journal of the American Oil Chemists' Society* 75(10):1417–20.

Codex Badianus. 1552. *An Aztec herbal: The classic codex of 1552*. Ed. and trans. William Gates, 2000. Mineola, N.Y.: Dover.

Codex Mendoza. 1542. Ed. Francisco del Paso y Troncoso, 1925. Mexico City: Museo Nacional de Arqueología, Historia y Etnografía.

Consensus Conference. 1985. Statement on lowering blood cholesterol to prevent heart disease. *Journal of the American Medical Association* 253:2080–86.

Conway, G. R., and E. B. Barbier. 1990. *After the green revolution: sustainable agriculture for development*. London: Earthscan Publications.

Cook, N. C., and S. Samaman. 1996. Flavonoids: chemistry, metabolism, cardio protective effects, and dietary sources. *Journal of Nutritional Biochemistry* 7:66–76.

Cooley, A. S. 1899. Athenas Polias on the Acropolis of Athens. *American Journal of Archaeology* 3(4–5):345–408.

Cordain, L. 1999. Cereal grains: humanity's double-edged sword. In Simopoulos, 1999b:19–73.

Cortés, H. 1522. *Carta de relación embiada a su sacra magestad del emperador nuestro señor por el capitán general de la Nueva España llamado D. Hernando Cortés*. Seville: Jacobo Rombreger Aleman. Reedited by Imprenta del Superior Gobierno del Brigadier José Antonio de Hogal, 1770. Mexico City.

Cortéz y Larraz, P. 1958. *Descripción geográfico-moral de la diócesis de Goathemala*. Vol. 20. Guatemala City: Sociedad de Geografía e Historia de Guatemala.

Cowan, C. W., and P. J. Watson. 1992. Introduction. In *The origins of agriculture: an international perspective*, ed. C. W. Cowan and P. J. Watson, 1–6. Washington, D.C.: Smithsonian Institution Press.

Craig-Schmidt, M. 1992. Fatty acids in foods. In Chow, 1992b:365–98.

Crawford, D. J. 1979. Food: tradition and change in Hellenistic Egypt. *World Archeology* 2(2):136–46.

Cuevas Sánchez, J. A. 1992. La agricultura tradicional en México: su importancia en la conservación de las plantas como recurso. In Universidad Autónoma Chapingo, 1992:91–97.

Cunnane, S. C., and L. U. Thompson, eds. 1995. *Flaxseed in human nutrition*. Champaign, Ill.: American Oil Chemists' Society Press.

Dabrowski, K., S. Czesny, and M. Matusiewicz. 2002. Coregonids. In Webster and Lim, 2002:230–44.

Demeyer, D., and M. Doreau. 1999. Targets and procedures for altering ruminant meat and milk lipids. *Proceedings of the Nutrition Society* 58:593–607.

Denke, M., and S. Grundy. 1992. Comparison on effects of lauric acid and palmitic acid on plasma lipids and lipoproteins. *American Journal of Clinical Nutrition* 56:895–98.

Department of Health. 1991. *Dietary reference values for food energy and nutrients for the U.K.* Report on Health and Social Subjects No. 41. Report of the Committee on Medical Aspects of Food Policy, London.

Dewailly, E., S. Bruneau, G. Lebel, P. Levallois, and J. P. Weber. 2001. Exposure of the Inuit population of Nunavik (Arctic, Québec) to lead and mercury. *Archives of Environmental Health* 56(4):350–57.

Díaz del Castillo, B. 1568. *La verdadera historia de la conquista de México*. Ed. J. Wright and J. Dead, 1800; trans. M. Keatinge. London.

Djousse, L., A. R. Folsom, M. A. Province, S. C. Hunt, and R. Curtis-Ellison. 2003. Dietary linolenic acid and carotid atherosclerosis: the National Heart, Lung, and Blood Institute family health study. *American Journal of Clinical Nutrition* 77:819–25.

Dominguez-Vazquez, G., B. Berlin, A. E. Castro Ramirez, and E. J. I. Estrada-Lugo. 2002. Revisión de la diversidad y patrones de distribución de Labiatae en Chiapas. *Anales del Instituto de Biología, Serie Botánica* 73(1):39–80.

Dowden, A. 2001. Fun and functional. Dot Pharmacy. 12 December. http://www.dotpharmacy.co.uk

Downey, R. K., G. Robbelen, and A. Ashri. 1989. Preface. In Robbelen, Downey, and Ashri, 1989:xvii–xviii.

Dressler, R. 1953. The pre-Columbian cultivated plants of Mexico. Harvard University, *Botanical Museum Leaflets* 16(6): 115–72.

Durán, D. 1570, 1579. *Historia de los indios de Nueva España e islas de la tierra firme*. 2 vols. Ed. A. M. Garibay, 1984. Mexico City: Biblioteca Porrua.

Dutton, H. J., and T. L. Mounts. 1966. Desaturation of fatty acids in seeds of higher plants. *Journal of Lipid Research* 7:221–25.

Dyerberg, J., H. O. Bang, E. Stoffersen, S. Moncada, and J. R. Vane. 1978. Eicosapentaenoic acid and prevention of thrombosis and atherosclerosis. *Lancet* 2:117–21.

Eaton, S. B., and S. B. Eaton III. 1999. Evolution, diet and health. Department of Anthropology and Radiology, Emory University, Atlanta, Ga., 12 pp.

———. 2000. Paleolithic vs. modern diets: selected pathophysiological implications. *European Journal of Nutrition* 39(2):67–70.

Eaton, S. B., S. B. Eaton III, and M. J. Konner. 1997. Paleolithic nutrition revisited: a twelve-year retrospective on its nature and implications. *European Journal of Nutrition* 51:207–16.

Eaton, S. B., S. B. Eaton III, M. J. Konner, and M. Shostak. 1996. An evolutionary perspective enhances understanding of human nutritional requirements. *Journal of Nutrition* 126:1732–40.

Eaton, S. B., S. B. Eaton III, A. J. Sinclair, L. Cordain, and N. J. Man. 1998. Dietary intake of long-chain polyunsaturated fatty acids during the Paleolithic. *World Review of Nutrition and Diet* 83:12–23.

Eaton, S. B., and M. J. Konner. 1985. Paleolithic nutrition: a consideration of its nature and current implications. *New England Journal of Medicine* 312:283–89.

Eckey, E. W. 1954. *Vegetable fats and oils.* American Chemical Society, Monograph Series. New York: Reinhold Publishing Corporation.

Economic Research Service. 2001. Diet, consumption, & health. United States Department of Agriculture. 10 December. http://www.ers.usda.gov

Emken, E. A. 1995. Trans-fatty acids and coronary heart disease risk: physicochemical properties, intake, and metabolism. *American Journal of Clinical Nutrition* 62(suppl.):659s–69s.

Emken, E. A., R. O. Adlof, and R. M. Gulley. 1994. Dietary linolenic acid influences desaturation and acylation of deuterium-labeled linoleic and linolenic acids in young adult males. *Biochimica et Biophysica Acta* 1213:277–88.

Engel, F. A. 1987. *De las begonias al maíz: vida y producción en el Perú antiguo.* Centro de Investigaciones de Zonas Aridas. Lima, Peru: Universidad Nacional Agraria La Molina.

Enser, M. 2000. Nutritional effects on meat flavor and stability. In Sim, Nakai, and Guenter, 2000:197–215.

Ershow, A., R. Nocolosi, and K. Hayes. 1981. Separation of the dietary fat and cholesterol influences on plasma lipoproteins of rhesus monkeys. *American Journal of Clinical Nutrition* 34:830–40.

Estilai, A., A. Hashemi, and K. Truman. 1990. Chromosome number and meiotic behavior of cultivated chia, *Salvia hispanica* (Lamiaceae). *HortScience* 25(12):1646–47.

Estrada Lugo, E. I. 1989. *El Códice Florentino: su información etnobotánica.* Chapingo, Mexico: Colegio de Postgraduados.

Estrada Lugo, I. J. 1992. Notas sobre la agricultura prehispánica en el *Códice Florentino.* In Universidad Autónoma Chapingo, 1992:69–77.

Ezaki, O., M. Takahashi, and T. Shigematsu. 1999. Long-term effects of dietary alpha-linolenic acid from perilla oil on serum fatty acids composition and on the risk factors of coronary heart disease in Japanese elderly subjects. *Journal of Nutritional Science and Vitaminology* 45(6):759–72.

Felger, R. S., and M. B. Moser. 1985. *People of the desert and sea: ethnobotany of the Seri Indians.* Tucson: University of Arizona Press.

Ferretti, A., and V. P. Flanagan. 1996. Anti tromboxane activity of dietary alpha-linolenic acid: a pilot study. *Prostaglandins, Leukotrienes and Essential Fatty Acids* 54(6):451–55.

Ferrier, L. K., L. Caston, S. Leeson, E. J. Squires, B. Celi, L. Thomas, and B. J. Holub. 1992. Changes in serum lipids and platelet fatty acid composition following consumption of eggs enriched in alpha-linolenic acid (LnA). *Food Research International* 25:263–68.

Ferro-Luzzi, A., and F. Branca. 1995. Mediterranean diet, Italian-style: prototype of a healthy diet. In Nestle, 1995b:1338s–45s.

Fick, G. N. 1988. Novel sunflower products and methods for their production: patent number 4,743,402. United States Patent, 12 pp.

Fieldsend, A. F., and J. I. L. Morison. 2000. Climatic conditions during seed growth significantly influence oil content and quality in winter and spring evening primrose crops (*Oenothera* spp.). *Industrial Crops and Products* 12:137–47.

Flax Council of Canada. 1996. Omega-3 in flax balance the diet. Conference of the Flax Council of Canada. 26 December 2001. http://www.flaxcouncil.ca/flaxnews1.htm

———. 2000. Flaxseed in egg production. 7 July. http://www.flaxcouncil.ca.

Floratech. 1996. FloraSun Nature shelf life success. International Flora Technologies, Inc., Gilbert, Ariz., 8 pp.

Food and Agricultural Policy Research Institute. 1995. *FAPRI 1995 U.S. agricultural outlook.* Iowa State University and University of Missouri-Columbia, Staff Report #1-95.

Food and Agriculture Organization. 1971. Energy and protein requirements. Report of a joint Food and Agriculture Organization/WHO ad hoc expert committee. Food and Nutritional Series, Food and Agriculture Organization, Rome.

———. 1994. *Fats and oils in human nutrition: report of a joint expert consultation.* Food and Nutrition Paper No. 57, Food and Agriculture Organization, Rome.

———. 1996. *World food summit.* Food and Agriculture Organization, Rome.

———. 2000a. *The state of food and agriculture.* Food and Agriculture Organization Agricultural Series, Rome.

———. 2000b. *The state of food insecurity in the world 2000.* Food and Agriculture Organization Agricultural Series, Rome.

———. 2001a. Food balance sheets. Food and Agriculture Organization stat

agriculture data. 12 October. http://apps.fao.org/page/collections?subset=
agriculture

————. 2001b. *The state of food and agriculture*. Food and Agriculture Organization
Agricultural Series, Rome.

Food and Drug Administration. 1999. GRAS notice No. GRN 000016. Center for
Food Safety and Applied Nutrition. 5 January 2002. http://www.cfsan.fda.gov/
~rdb/opa-g016.html

————. 2000. Food labeling: health claims and labeling statements; dietary fiber
and cancer; antioxidant vitamins and cancer; omega-3 fatty acids and coronary
heart disease; folate and neural tube defects; revocation. 21 CFR Part 101 (docket
nos. 91N-0101, 91N-0098, 91N-0103, and 91N-100H) RIN 0910-AA19. Final rule.
22 December 2001. http://www.cfsan.fda.gov/~lrd/fr001003.html

————. 2001. FDA announces advisory on methyl mercury in fish. Food and Drug
Administration Talk Paper TO1-04. 5 January 2002. http://www.fda.gov/bbs/
topics/ANSWERS/2001/ANS01065.html

Food Engineering International. 1997. Functional food in Europe. 22 August 2000.
http://www.broste.com/food/lib/FunctionalFood.htm

Food Safety Authority of Ireland. 2002. Summary of investigation of dioxins, furans
and PCBs in farmed salmon, wild salmon, farmed trout and fish oil capsules.
21 March 2002. http://www.fsai.ie/pressreleases_index.htm

Forse, R. A., ed. 1994. *Diet, nutrition, and immunity*. Boca Raton, Fla.: CRC Press.

Freese, R., and M. Mutanen. 1997. Alpha-linolenic acid and marine long-chain n-
3 fatty acids differ only slightly in their effects on hemostatic factors in healthy
subjects. *American Journal of Clinical Nutrition* 66:591–98.

Fry, J. L., P. Van Walleghem, P. W. Waldroup, and R. H. Harms. 1965. Fish meal
studies: effects of levels and sources of fishy flavor in broiler meat. *Poultry Science*
44:1016–19.

Fu, Z., and A. J. Sinclair. 2000. Novel pathway of metabolism of alpha-linolenic acid
in the guinea pig. *Pediatric Research* 47(3):414–17.

Galli, C., and A. P. Simopoulos, eds. 1988. *Dietary omega-3 and omega-6 fatty acids*.
NATO ASI Series No. 171. New York: Plenum Press and NATO Scientific Affairs
Division.

García-Closas, R., C. A. González, A. Agudo, and E. Riboli. 1999. Intake of specific
carotenoids and flavonoids and the risk of gastric cancer in Spain. *Cancer Causes
and Control* 10:71–75.

García Cook, A. 1992. Sobre el origen de la agricultura en México. In Universidad
Autónoma Chapingo, 1992:3–11.

García de Palacio, D. 1583. Carta relación de Diego García de Palacio a Felipe II sobre
la provincia de Guatemala, 8 de marzo de 1576. Ed. Pedro de Ocharte, Mexico,
reedited by Gráficas Ultra, 1944. Madrid.

Garibay, A. M. 1989. Introdución al décimo libro. In *Historia general de las cosas de Nueva España* by B. de Sahagún, 1579. Ed. A. M. Garibay. Mexico City: Editorial Porrua.

Garn, S. M., and W. R. Leónard. 1989. What did our ancestors eat? *Nutrition Reviews* 47:337–45.

Garrison, R. H., and E. Somer. 1990. *The nutrition desk reference.* New Canaan, Conn.: Keats Publishing.

Gatlin, D. M. 2002. Red drum, *Sciaenops ocellatus.* In Webster and Lim, 2002:147–58.

Gil, M. 1975. Supplies of oil in medieval Egypt: a Geniza study. *Journal of Near Eastern Studies* 34(1):63–73.

GISSI. 1999. Dietary supplementation with n-3 polyunsaturated fatty acids and vitamin E after myocardial infarction: results of the GISSI-Prevenzione trial. *Lancet* 354:447–55.

Glew, R. H., Y. S. Huang, T. A. Vander Jagt, L. T. Chuang, S. K. Bhatti, M. A. Magnussen, and D. J. Vander Jagt. 2001. Fatty acid composition of the milk lipids of Nepalese women: correlation between fatty acid composition of serum phospholipids and melting point. *Prostaglandins, Leukotrienes and Essential Fatty Acids* 65(3):147–56.

Gomez Pompa, A. 1993. Las raíces de la etnobotánica mexicana. In *Logros y perspectivas del conocimiento de los recursos vegetales de México en vísperas del siglo XXI*, ed. S. Guevara, P. Moreno Casasola, and J. Rzedowski, 26–37. Mexico City: Instituto de Ecología y Sociedad Botánica de México.

González, J. 1581. *Relación de Xonotla.* Sección indiferente general, legajo 1529, Archivo General de Indias, Seville, Spain. 30 October 2001. http://mlab.uiah.fi/simultaneous/text/Project.html

González-Esquerra, R., and S. Leeson. 2000. Effects of menhaden oil and flaxseed in broiler diets on sensory quality and lipid composition of poultry meat. *British Poultry Science* 41(4):481–88.

Gortari, E. de. 1979. *La ciencia en la historia de México.* Mexico City: Grijalbo.

Government Services Canada, 2001. *Functional foods and nutraceuticals: market, industry and distribution.* Ottawa: Public Work and Government Services Canada, Canadian Government Publishing Directorate.

Griffin, B. A. 1999. Lipoprotein atherogenicity: an overview of current mechanisms. *Proceedings of the Nutrition Society* 58:163–69.

Griffin, H. D. 1992. Manipulation of egg yolk cholesterol: a physiologist's view. *World's Poultry Science Journal* 48:103–12.

Grillo, B., O. Rampoldi, C. Servetto, E. López, R. Hermo, and W. Alallon. 1999. Efecto de una dieta enriquecida con krill sobre la composición de ácidos grasos del huevo de gallina. *Clínica e Investigación en Arteriosclerosis* 2(1):16–18.

Gumprecht, B. 2001. *The Los Angeles River*. Baltimore, Md.: Johns Hopkins University Press.

Grundy, S. M. 1986. Comparison of monounsaturated fatty acids and carbohydrates for lowering plasma cholesterol. *New England Journal of Medicine* 314(12):745–48.

———. 1997. What is the desirable ratio of saturated, polyunsaturated, and monounsaturated fatty acids in the diet? In *Fats and oil consumption in health and disease*, ed. R. S. Rivlin. *Proceedings of a symposium held at the Rockefeller University, New York. American Journal of Clinical Nutrition* 66(4s):988–90.

Grundy, S. M., E. Barrett-Connor, and L. L. Rudel. 1988. Workshop on the impact of dietary cholesterol on plasma lipoproteins and atherogenesis. *Arterioclerosis* 8:95–101.

Guallar, E., A. Aro, F. J. Jiménez, J. M. Martín-Moreno, I. Salminen, P. van't Veer, A. F. M. Kardinaal, J. Gomez-Aracena, B. C. Martin, L. Kohlmeier, J. D. Kark, V. P. Mazaev, J. Ringstad, J. Guillen, R. A. Riemersma, J. K. Huttunen, M. Thamm, and F. J. Kok. 1999. Omega-3 fatty acids in adipose tissue and risk of myocardial infarction: the EURAMIC study. *Arteriosclerosis, Thrombosis and Vascular Biology* 19:1111–18.

Hagemann, M., F. R. Earle, and I. A. Wolff. 1968. Search for new industrial oils. XIV. Seed oils of Labiatae. *Lipids* 2(5):371–80.

Hansen, J. C. 2000. Environmental contaminants and human health in the Arctic. *Toxicology Letters* 112–13:119–25.

Hansen, T. K., C. Bindsley-Jensen, P. S. Skov, and L. K. Poulsen. 1997. Codfish allergy in adults: IgE cross-reactivity among fish species. *Annals of Allergy, Asthma and Immunology* 78:187–94.

Hardin, J. O., J. L. Milligan, and V. D. Sidwell. 1964. The influence of solvent extracted fish meal and stabilized fish oil in broiler rations on performance and on the flavor of broiler meat. *Poultry Science* 43:858–60.

Hardy, R. W. 2002. Rainbow trout, *Oncorhynchus mykiss*. In Webster and Lim, 2002:184–202.

Harel, Z., S. Riggs, R. Vaz, L. W. Menzies, and G. Menzies. 2001. Omega-3 polyunsaturated fatty acids in adolescents: knowledge and consumption. *Journal of Adolescent Health* 28(1):10–15.

Hargis, P. S. 1988. Modifying egg yolk cholesterol in the domestic fowl: a review. *World's Poultry Science Journal* 44:15–29.

Harlan, J. R. 1992. *Crops and man*. Madison, Wis.: American Society of Agronomy and Crop Science Society of America.

Hashim, M. Y. 1996. The world's largest palm oil producer. *USA Today/International Edition*, special advertising section, 26 April:7b.

Hasler, C. M. 2000. The changing face of functional foods. *Journal of the American College of Nutrition* 19(5):499s–506s.

Hassel, C. A., E. A. Mensing, and D. G. Gallaher. 1997. Dietary stearic aid reduces plasma and hepatic cholesterol concentrations without increasing bile acid excretion in cholesterol-fed hamsters. *Journal of Nutrition* 127:1148–55.

Hawkes, J. G. 1998. The introduction of New World crops into Europe after 1492. In *Plants for food and medicine*, ed. H. D. V. Prendergast, N. L. Etkin, D. R. Harris, and P. J. Houghton, 147–59. Kew, U.K.: Board of Trustees of the Royal Botanic Gardens.

Hebert, P., N. Fiebach, K. Eberlein, J. Taylor, and C. Hennekens. 1988. The community-based randomized trials of pharmacological treatment of mild-to-moderate hypertension. *American Journal of Epidemiology* 127:581–90.

Hebling, A., M. L. McCants, J. J. Musmand, H. J. Schwartz, and S. B. Lehrer. 1996. Immune-pathogenesis of fish allergy: identification of fish-allergic adults by skin test and radioallergsorbent test. *Annals of Allergy, Asthma and Immunology* 77:48–54.

Hegsted, D. M., R. B. McGandy, M. L. Myers, and F. J. Stare. 1965. Quantitative effects of dietary fat on serum cholesterol in man. *American Journal of Clinical Nutrition* 17:281–95.

Heil, C. 1995. The pre-Columbian lacquer of West Mexico. *Neara Journal* 30 (1–2):32–39.

Helm, P. A., T. F. Bidleman, G. A. Stern, and K. Koczanski. 2002. Polychlorinated naphthalenes and coplanar polychlorinated biphenyls in beluga whale (*Delphinapterus leucas*) and ringed seal (*Phoca hispida*) from the eastern Canadian Arctic. *Environmental Pollution* 119:60–78.

Helsing, E. 1995. Traditional diets and disease patterns of the Mediterranean, circa 1960. In Nestle, 1995b:1329s–37s.

Hennekens, C., and J. Buring. 1985. Smoking and coronary disease in women. *Journal of the American Medical Association* 253: 3003–4.

Hennekens, C. H., J. E. Buring, and S. L. Mayrent. 1990. Clinical and epidemiological data on the effects of fish oil in cardio-vascular disease. In Lees and Karel, 1990:71–85.

Herber, S. M., and M. E. Van Elswyk. 1996. Dietary marine algae promotes efficient deposition of n-3 fatty acids for the production of enriched shell eggs. *Poultry Science* 75:1501–7.

Hernández, E. 1985. Biología agrícola: los conocimientos biológicos y su aplicación a la agricultura. Mexico City: CECSA.

———. 1993. Aspects of plant domestication in Mexico: a personal view. In Ramamoorthy et al., 1993:733–77.

Hernández, F. 1575. *Antigüedades de la Nueva España*. Ed. A. H. de León Portilla, 1986. Madrid: Información y Revistas SA.

———. 1576. Materia medicinal de la Nueva España.

Hernández-Bermejo, J. E., and J. León. 1992. Cultivos marginados: otra perspectiva. Food and Agriculture Organization, Colección Food and Agriculture Organization, Producción y Protección Vegetal No. 26, Rome.

Hernández Gómez, J. A. 1994. Chía (*Salvia hispanica*): antecedentes y prespectivas en México. In *Primer simposium internacional sobre etnobotánica en Mesoamérica*, ed. J. A. Cuevas Sánchez, E. Estrada Lugo, and E. Cedillo Portugal, 173–80. Chapingo, Mexico: Universidad Autónoma Chapingo.

Hertog, M. G., D. Kromhout, and C. Aravanis. 1995. Flavonoid intake and long-term risk of coronary heart disease and cancer in the seven countries study. *Archives of Internal Medicine* 155(4):381–86.

Hertog, M. G., E. J. Feskens, P. C. Hollman, M. B. Katan, and D. Kromhout. 1993. Dietary antioxidant flavonoids and risk of coronary heart disease: the Zutphen elderly study. *Lancet* 342(8878):1007–11.

Hertog, M. G. L., and P. C. H. Hollman. 1996. Potential health effects of the dietary flavonol quercetin. *European Journal of Clinical Nutrition* 50:63–71.

Herzlich, B. C., E. Lichstein, N. Schulhoff, M. Weinstock, M. Pagala, K. Ravindran, T. Namba, F. Nieto, S. Stabler, R. Allen, and M. Malinow. 1996. Relationship among homocyst(e)ine, vitamin B-12 and cardiac disease in the elderly: association between vitamin B-12 deficiency and decreased left ventricular ejection fraction. *Journal of Nutrition* 126:1249s–53s.

Hicks, S. 1966. *Desert plants and people*. San Antonio, Tex.: Naylor Company.

Hirovonen, T., P. Pietinen, M. Virtanen, M. L. Ovaskainen, S. Hakkinen, D. Albanes, and J. Virtamo. 2001. Intake of flavonols and flavones and risk of coronary heart disease in male smokers. *Epidemiology* 12(1):62–67.

Hites, R. A., J. A. Foran, D. O. Carpenter, M. C. Hamilton, B. A. Knuth, and S. J. Schwager. 2004. Global assessment of organic contaminants in farmed salmon. *Science* 303:226–29.

Holdas, A., and K. N. May. 1966. Fish oil and fishy flavor of eggs and carcasses of hens. *Poultry Science* 45:1405–7.

Hollingsworth, P. 2000. Marketing trends fueling healthful foods success. *Foodtechnology* 54(10):53–59.

Holman, R. T., M. M. Mahfouz, L. D. Lawson, and E. G. Hill. 1994. Metabolic effects of isomeric octadecenoic acids. In *Dietary fats and health*, ed. E. G. Perkins and W. J. Visek, 320–42. Champaign, Ill.: American Oil Chemists' Society Press.

Homer, P., and P. J. Schaible. 1980. *Poultry: feeds and nutrition*. Westport, Conn.: AVI Publishing, USA.

Horrobin, D. F. 1988. Polyunsaturated oils of marine and plant origins and their uses in clinical medicine. In Galli and Simopoulos, 1988:297–350.

Horrocks, L. A., and Y. K. Yeo. 2000. Docosahexaenoic acid—enriched foods: production of eggs and health benefits. In Sim, Nakai, and Guenter, 2000:173–80.

Howard, B. V., J. S. Hannah, C. C. Heiser, K. A. Jablonski, M. C. Paidi, L. Alarif, D. C. Robbins, and W. J. Howard. 1995. Polyunsaturated fatty acids result in greater cholesterol lowering and less triacylglycerol elevation than do monounsaturated fatty acids in a dose-response comparison in a multiracial study group. *American Journal of Clinical Nutrition* 62:392–402.

Howell, R. W., and F. I. Collins. 1957. Factors affecting linolenic and linoleic acid content of soybean. *Agronomy Journal* 49:593–97.

Hu, F. B., M. J. Stampfer, J. E. Manson, E. B. Rimm, A. Wolk, G. A. Colditz, C. H. Hennekens, and W. C. Willet. 1999. Dietary intake of alpha-linolenic acid and risk of fatal ischemic heart disease among women. *American Journal of Clinical Nutrition* 69:890–97.

Huang, Y. S., and A. J. Sinclair, eds. 1998. *Lipids in infant nutrition*. Champaign, Ill.: American Oil Chemists' Society Press.

Hulan, H. W., R. G. Ackman, W. M. N. Ratanayake, and F. G. Proudfoot. 1988. Omega-3 fatty acid levels and general performance of commercial broilers fed practical levels of redfish meal. *Poultry Science* 68:153–62.

———. 1989. Omega-3 fatty acid levels and performance of commercial broilers fed practical levels of redfish meal. *Canadian Journal of Animal Science* 68:533–47.

Hunter, J. E. 1988. Omega-3 fatty acids from vegetable oil. In Galli and Simopoulos, 1988:43–56.

Illingworth, D. R., and D. Ullmann. 1990. Effects of omega-3 fatty acids on risk factors for cardiovascular disease. In Lees and Karel, 1990:39–69.

INIFAP. 1995. *Informe nacional para la conferencia técnica internacional de la FAO sobre los recursos fitogenéticos*. Mexico City: Instituto Nacional de Investigaciones Forestales y Agropecuarias.

Innis, S. M., and R. Dyer. 1997. Dietary triacylglycerols with palmitic acid (16:0) in the 2-position increase plasma and chylomicron triacylglycerols, but reduce phospholipid arachidonic and docosahexaenoic acids, and alter cholesteryl ester metabolism in formula-fed piglets. *Journal of Nutrition* 127:1311–19.

Innis, S. M., and D. J. King. 1999. Trans-fatty acids in human milk are inversely associated with concentrations of essential all-cis -6 and n-3 fatty acids in plasma lipids of breast-fed infants. *American Journal of Clinical Nutrition* 70:383–90.

Instituto Nacional de Alimentos. 2003. *Análisis físico-químico de semillas de chía*. Buenos Aires, 1 p.

International Flora Technologies, Inc. 1990. *Oil of chia*. Apache Junction, Ariz., 2 pp.

International Life Science Institute. 1999. North America food component reports. *Critical Reviews in Food Science and Nutrition* 39:203–316.

Iso, H., K. M. Raxrode, M. J. Stampfer, J. E. Manson, G. A. Colditz, F. E. Speizer, H. Hennekens, and W. Willet. 2001. Intake of fish oil and omega-3 fatty acids and risk of stroke in women. *Journal of the American Medical Association* 285(3):304–12.

Jacobs, M., J. Ferrario J., and C. Byrne. 2002. Investigation of polychlorinated dibenzo-p-dioxins, dibenzo-p-furans and selected coplanar biphenyls in Scottish farmed Atlantic salmon (*Salmo salar*). *Chemosphere* 47(2):183–91.

Jacobsen, C., J. A. Nissen, and A. S. Meyer. 1999. Effect of ascorbic acid on iron release from the emulsifier interface and on the oxidative flavor deterioration in fish oil enriched mayonnaise. *Journal of Agricultural and Food Chemistry* 47:4917–26.

Jacobsen, C., M. Timm, and A. S. Meyer. 2001. Oxidation in fish oil enriched mayonnaise: ascorbic acid and low pH increase oxidative deterioration. *Journal of Agricultural and Food Chemistry* 49:3947–56.

James, J. M., R. M. Helm, A. W. Burks, and S. B. Leherer. 1997. Comparison of pediatric and adult IgE antibody binding to fish proteins. *Annals of Allergy, Asthma and Immunology* 79:131–37.

James, W. P. T. 1995. Nutrition science and policy research: implications for Mediterranean diets. In Nestle, 1995b:1324s–28s.

Jenkins, D. J. A., A. L. Jenkins, T. M. S. Wolever, and V. Vuksan. 1994. Fiber and physiological and potentially therapeutic effects of slowing carbohydrate absorption. In *New developments in dietary fiber: physiological, physicochemical and analytical aspects*, ed. I. Furda and J. Brine, 129–34. New York: Plenum Press.

Jensen, C. L., M. Maude, R. E. Anderson, and W. C. Heird. 2000. Effect of docosahexaenoic acid supplementation of lactating women on the fatty acid composition of breast milk lipids and maternal and infant plasma phospholipids. *American Journal of Clinical Nutrition* 71(suppl.):292s–99s.

Jensen, R. G. 1992. Fatty acids in milk and dairy products. In Chow, 1992b:95–135.

Jensen, R. G., and C. L. Lammi-Keefe. 1998. Current status of research on the composition of bovine and human milk lipids. In Huang and Sinclair, 1998:168–91.

Jiang, Y. H., R. B. McGeachin, and C. A. Bailey. 1994. Alpha-tocopherol, beta-carotene and retinol enrichment of chicken eggs. *Poultry Science* 73:1137–43.

Jiménez-Escrig, A., I. Jiménez-Jiménez, R. Pulido, and F. Saura-Calixto. 2001. Antioxidant activity of fresh and processed edible seaweeds. *Journal of the Science of Food and Agriculture* 81:530–34.

Jones, P., B. R. Toy, and M. C. Cha. 1994. Differential fatty acid accretion in heart, liver and adipose tissues of rats fed beef tallow, fish oil, olive oil and safflower oils at three levels of energy intake. *American Institute of Nutrition* 125:1175–82.

Judd, J. T., B. A. Clevidence, R. A. Muesing, J. Wittes, M. E. Sunkin, and J. J. Podczasy. 1994. Dietary trans-fatty acids: effects on plasma lipids and lipoproteins of healthy men and women. *American Journal of Clinical Nutrition* 59:861–68.

Karleskind, A., and J. P. Wolff, eds. 1996. *Oils and fats manual.* Vol. 1. Paris: Lavoisier.

Kashambuzi, E. 1999. *The paradox of hunger and abundance*. Orlando, Fla.: Rivercross Publishing.

Katan, M., P. Zock, and R. Mensink. 1995. Dietary oils, serum lipoproteins, and coronary heart disease. *American Journal of Clinical Nutrition* 61(suppl.):1368s–73s.

Katan, M. B. 1990. Health effects of dietary fatty acids. In Bont, 1990:10–15.

Keli, S. O., M. G. Hertog, E. J. Feskens, and D. Kromhout. 1996. Dietary flavonoids, antioxidant vitamins, and incidence of stroke: the Zutphen study. *Archives of Internal Medicine* 156(6):637–42.

Kelly, D. S. 1999. Fatty acids and immune functions. In *Military strategies for sustainment of nutrition and immune function in the field*, ed. Committee on Military Nutrition Research, Food and Nutrition Board and Institute of Medicine, 305–16. Washington, D.C.: National Academy Press.

Keys, A. J., J. T. Anderson, and F. Grande. 1965. Serum cholesterol response to changes in the diet. IV. Particular saturated fatty acids in the diet. *Metabolism* 1:776–87.

Kirchhoff, P. 1943. Mesoamérica. *Acta Americana* 1:92–107.

KLSE Stock Market. 2001. LTKM—omega 3 egg producer, 8 percent dividend on 4 September. Asiaco.com. 25 January. http://forum.asiaco.com/stockmarket/428.shtml

Knekt, P., R. Jarvinen, A. Reunanen, and J. Maatela. 1996. Flavonoid intake and coronary mortality in Finland: a cohort study. *British Medical Journal* 312(7029):478–81.

Knekt, P., R. Jarvinen, R. Seppanen, M. Hellovaara, L. Teppo, E. Pukkala, and A. Aromaa. 1997. Dietary flavonoids and the risk of lung cancer and other malignant neoplasms. *American Journal of Epidemiology* 146(3):223–30.

Koeheler, H. H., and G. E. Bearse. 1975. Egg flavour quality as affected by fish meals or fish oils in laying rations. *Poultry Science* 54:881–89.

Krauss, R. M., R. H. Eckel, B. Howard, L. J. Appel, S. R. Daniels, R. J. Deckelbaum, J. W. Erdman, P. Kris-Etherton, I. J. Goldberg, T. A. Kotchen, A. H. Lichtenstein, W. E. Mitch, R. Mullis, K. Robinson, J. Wylie-Rosett, S. S. Jeor, J. Suttie, D. L. Tribble, and T. L. Bazarre. 2000. AHA dietary guidelines. Revision 2000: a statement for healthcare professionals from the Nutrition Committee of the American Heart Association. *Circulation* 102:2284–99.

Kromhout, D., E. B. Bosschieter, and C. de Lezenne Coulander. 1985. The inverse relation between fish consumption and 20-year mortality from coronary heart disease. *New England Journal of Medicine* 312:1205–9.

Kung, T. K., and F. A. Kummerow. 1950. The deposition of linolenic acid in chickens fed linseed oil. *Poultry Science* 29:846–51.

Kweon, M. H., H. J. Hwang, and H. C. Sung. 2001. Identification and antioxidant activity of novel chlorogenic acid derivatives from bamboo (*Phyllostachys edulis*). *Journal of Agricultural and Food Chemistry* 49:4646–55.

Kwok, T., J. Woo, S. Ho, and A. Sham. 2000. Vegetarianism and ischemic heart disease in older Chinese women. *Journal of the American College of Nutrition* 19(5):622–27.

Lands, W. E. 1992. Biochemistry and physiology of n-3 acids. *Federation of American Societies for Experimental Biology* 6:2530–36.

Las Casas, B. de. 1552. *Brevísima relación de la destrucción de las Indias*. Ed. Ediciones 29, 1997. Barcelona: BIGSA.

Lauritzen, L., H. S. Hansen, M. H. Jorgensen, and K. F. Michaelson. 2001. The essentiality of long-chain n-3 fatty acids in relation to development and function of the brain and retina. *Progress in Lipid Research* 40:1–94.

Leaf, A. 2002. On the reanalysis of the GISS-prevenzione. *Circulation* 105(16):1874–75.

Leaf, A., and P. C. Weber. 1987. A new era for science in nutrition. *American Journal of Clinical Nutrition* 45:1048–53.

Le Conseil d'Etat. 1973. Interdiction de l'huile de lin. *Journal Officiel*, 1523–26.

Lee, K. H., J. M. Olomu, and J. S. Sim. 1991. Live performance, carcass yield, protein, and energy retention of broiler chickens fed canola and flax full-fat seeds and the restored mixtures of meal and oil. *Canadian Journal of Animal Science* 71:897–903.

Lees, R. S., and M. Karel. 1990. *Omega-3 fatty acids in health and disease*. New York: Marcel Dekker.

León Portilla, M. 1966. *La filosofía nahuatl estudiada en sus fuentes*. Mexico City: Instituto de Investigaciones Históricas, Universidad Nacional Autónoma.

———. 1971. *De Teotihuacán a los aztecas: antología de fuentes e interpretaciones históricas*. Mexico City: Instituto de Investigaciones Históricas, Universidad Nacional Autónoma.

———. 1988. *Los antiguos mexicanos: a través de sus crónicas y cantares*. Mexico City: Fondo de Cultura Económica.

Lessire, M., M. Doreau, and A. Aumaitre. 1996. Digestive and metabolic utilization of fats in domestic animals. In Karleskind and Wolff, 1996:703–13.

Lewis, C. E., and J. O. McGee. 1992. Natural killer cells in tumour biology. In *The natural killer cells*, ed. C. E. Lewis and J. O. McGee, 175–203. Oxford: Oxford University Press.

Lewis, N. M., K. Schalch, and S. E. Scheideler. 1998. Incorporation of omega-3 fatty acid—enriched eggs in low fat diets of hypercholerolemic humans. In Simopoulos, 1998b:24–37.

Li, D., A. Sinclair, A. Wilson, S. Nakkote, F. Kelly, L. Abedin, N. Mann, and

A. Turner. 1999. Effect of dietary alpha-linolenic acid on thrombotic risk factors in vegetarian men. *American Journal of Clinical Nutrition* 69:872–82.

Lichtenstein, A. H. 1999. Dietary fat: a history. *Nutrition Reviews* 57(1):11–14.

Liepa, G. U., and M. A. Gorman. 1991. Nutritional and health aspects of dietary lipids. In *Introduction to fats and oils technology*, ed. P. J. Wan, 321–30. Champaign, Ill.: American Oil Chemists' Society Press.

Lim, Ch., I. G. Borlongan, and F. P. Pascual. 2002. Milkfish, *Chanos chanos*. In Webster and Lim, 2002:172–83.

Lin, K. Y., and J. R. Daniel. 1994. Structure of chia seed polysaccharide exudate. *Carbohydrate Polymers* (23):13–18.

Lin, K. Y., J. R. Daniel, and R. L. Whistler. 1994. Structure of chia seed polysaccharide exudate. *Carbohydrate Polymers* 23:13–18.

Lin, L. J. 1996. FDA considering GRAS status for Solin. *INFORM* 7(6):640.

Lobb, K. 1992. Fatty acid classification and nomenclature. In Chow, 1992b:1–45.

López-Ferrer, S., M. D. Baucells, A. C. Barroeta, and M. A. Grashorn. 1999. N-3 enrichment of chicken meat using fish oil: alternative substitution with rapeseed and linseed oils. *Poultry Science* 78:356–65.

Lorenzana, F. A. 1770. Documentos y notas introductorias. In *Carta de relación embiada a su Sacra Magestad del Emperador Nuestro Señor por el Capitán General de la Nueva España llamado D. Fernando Cortés*. Mexico City: Imprenta del Superior Gobierno del Brigadier D. Joseph Antonio de Hogal.

Lorgeril, M. de, S. Renaud, N. Mamelle, P. Salen, J. L. Martin, I. Monjaud, J. Guidollet, P. Touboul, and J. Delaye. 1994. Mediterranean alpha-linolenic acid-rich diet in secondary prevention of coronary heart disease. *Lancet* 343:1454–59.

Lorgeril, M. de, P. Salen, J. L. Martin, N. Mamelle, I. Monjaud, P. Touboui, and J. Delaye. 1996. Effect of a Mediterranean type of diet on the rate of cardiovascular complications in patients with coronary artery disease. *Journal of the American College of Cardiology* 28(5):103–5.

Loria, R. M., and D. A. Padgett. 1997. Alpha-linolenic acid prevents the hypercholesteremic effects of cholesterol addition to a corn oil diet. *Nutritional Biochemistry* 8:140–46.

Lozoya, X. 1990. Presentación. In *Primera y segunda y tercera partes de la historia medicinal de las cosas que se traen de nuestras Indias Occidentales* by N. Monardes, 1574. Ed. E. Denot and N. Satanowsky. Mexico City: Instituto Mexicano de Seguro Social.

Lucena, M. 1992. *Así vivián los aztecas*. Madrid: Editorial Anaya.

MacLaren, J., and Y. Sugiura. 1991. The demise of the fifth sun. In *Seeds of change: a quincentennial commemoration*, ed. H. J. Viola and C. Margolis, 17–41. Washington, D.C.: Smithsonian Institution Press.

Madhusudhan, K. T., H. P. Ramesh, T. Ogawa, K. Sasaoka, and N. Singh. 1986. Detoxification of commercial linseed meal for use in broiler rations. *Poultry Science* 65:164–71.

Madsen, C. 1997. Prevalence of food allergy intolerance in Europe. *Environmental Toxicology and Pharmacology* 4:163–67.

Mah, P. 2000. Functional foods and nutraceuticals: the new frontier. Canadian Functional Food Network, Alberta Economic Development. 17 March. http://www.agric.gov.ab.ca/marketnews/functional2000-html/

Makris, D. P., and J. T. Rossiter. 2001. Comparison of quercetin and a non-orthohydroxy flavonol as antioxidant by competing in vitro oxidation reactions. *Journal of Agricultural and Food Chemistry* 49:3370–77.

Malinow, M. R. 1996. Plasma homocyst(e)ine: a risk factor for arterial occlusive diseases. *Journal of Nutrition* 126:1238s–43s.

Mantzioris, E., L. G. Cleland, R. A. Gibson, M. A. Neumann, M. Demasi, and M. J. James. 2000. Biochemical effects of a diet containing foods enriched with n-3 fatty acids. *American Journal of Clinical Nutrition* 72:42–48.

Mantzioris, E., M. J. James, R. A. Gibson, and L. G. Cleland. 1995. Differences exist in the relationships between dietary linoleic and alpha-linolenic acids and their respective long-chain metabolites. *American Journal of Clinical Nutrition* 61:320–24.

Marlett, J. A., K. B. Hosig, N. W. Vollendorf, F. L. Shinnik, V. S. Haack, and J. A. Story. 1994. Mechanism of serum cholesterol reduction by oat bran. *Hepatology* 20:1450–57.

Marshall, A. C., K. S. Kubena, K. R. Hinton, P. S. Hargis, and M. E. Van Elswyk. 1994. N-3 fatty acid enriched table eggs: a survey of consumer acceptability. *Poultry Science* 73:1334–40.

Marshall, A. C., A. R. Sams, and M. E. Van Elswyk. 1994. Oxidative stability and sensory quality of stored eggs from hens fed 1.5 percent menhaden oil. *Journal of Food Science* 59(3):561–63.

Martínez, M. 1994. *Catálogo de nombres vulgares y científicos de plantas mexicanas*. Mexico City: Fondo de Cultura Económica.

Martínez Arevalo, J. V. 1996. *Informe nacional para la conferencia técnica internacional de la FAO sobre los recursos fitogenéticos*. Guatemala City: Gobierno de Guatemala, 58 pp.

Masumoto, T. 2002. Yellowtail, *Seriola quinqueradiata*. In Webster and Lim, 2002:131–46.

Masuoka, S. 2001. Marta's mission. Asociación Mexicana de Arte y Cultura Popular. 10 November. http://amacup.org.mx/amacup.html

Matos Moctezuma, E. 1989. *The Aztecs*. New York: Rizzoli.

———. 1994. *The great temple of the Aztecs: treasures of Tenochtitlan*. New York: Thames and Hudson.

Mattson, F., and S. M. Grundy. 1985. Comparison of the effects of dietary saturated, monounsaturated, and polyunsaturated fatty acids on plasma lipids and lipoproteins in man. *Journal of Lipid Research* 26:194–202.

Mayerson, P. 1997. The role of flax in Roman and Fatimid Egypt. *Journal of Near Eastern Studies* 56(3):201–7.

Mazza, G., and B. D. Oomah. 1995. Flaxseed, dietary fiber, and cyanogens. In Cunnane and Thompson, 1995:56–81.

McAllister, D. 1999. *Consumer attitudes on eggs and omega 3 enrichment*. Market Research Report prepared by McAllister Consulting, Antrim, Northern Ireland.

McBride, J. 1999. A snapshot of blood homocysteine levels. 6 October. http://www.ars.usda.gov/is/AR/archive/mar99/snap0399.htm

McCaa, R. 1995. Fue el siglo XVI una catástrofe demográfica para México? Una respuesta basada en la demografía histórica no cuantitativa. *Cuadernos de Historia* 15:123–36.

McClung de Tapia, E. 1997. La domesticación del maíz. *Antropología Mexicana* 5(25):34–39.

McDougall, J., K. Litzau, E. Haver, V. Saunders, and G. A. Spiller. 1995. Rapid reduction of serum cholesterol and blood pressure by twelve-day, very low fat, strictly vegetarian diet. *Journal of the American College of Nutrition* 14(5):491–96.

McGuire, S. O., D. W. Alexander, and K. L. Fritsche. 1997. Fish oil source differentially affects rat immune cell alpha-tocopherol concentration. *Journal of Nutrition* 127:1388–94.

McKinlay, M. C. 2000. Nutritional aspects and possible pathological mechanisms of hyperhomocysteinaemia: an independent risk factor for vascular disease. *Proceedings of the Nutrition Society* 59:221–37.

McLennan, P. L. 1993. Relative effects of dietary saturated, monounsaturated, and polyunsaturated fatty acids on cardiac arrhythmias in rats. *American Journal of Clinical Nutrition* 57:207–12.

McLennan, P. L., and J. A. Dallimore. 1994. Dietary canola oil modifies myocardial fatty acids and inhibits cardiac arrhythmias in rats. *American Journal of Clinical Nutrition* 125:1003–5.

Mensink, R., and M. Katan. 1992. Effect of dietary fatty acids on serum lipids and lipoproteins: a meta-analysis of 27 trials. *Arteriosclerosis, Thrombosis and Vascular Biology* 12:911–19.

Mensink, R. P., and M. B. Katan. 1990. Effect of dietary trans-fatty acids on high density and low density lipoprotein cholesterol in healthy subjects. *New England Journal of Medicine* 323:439–45.

Miller, A. A. 1975. *Climatología*. Barcelona: Ediciones Omega SA.

Miller, D., and P. Robisch. 1969. Comparative effect of herring, menhaden, and safflower oils on broiler tissues fatty acid composition and flavor. *Poultry Science* 48:2146–57.

Mingione, E., and E. Pugliese. 1994. Rural subsistence, migration, urbanization, and the new global food regime. In *From Columbus to Conagra: the globalization of agriculture and food*, ed. A. Bonanno, L. Busch, W. Friedland, L. Gouveia, and E. Mingione, 52–68. Lawrence: University Press of Kansas.

Miranda, S. 1978. Evolución de cultivares nativos de México. *Ciencia y Desarrollo* 3(21):130–31.

Moldenke, H. N., and A. L. Moldenke. 1986. *Plants of the Bible*. Mineola, N.Y.: Dover.

Molins Fábrega, N. 1955. El códice Mendocino y la economía de Tenochtitlán. *Revista Mexicana de Estudios Antropológicos* 14:303–35.

Molketin, K., and D. Precht. 1995. Determination of trans-octadecenoic acids in German margarines, shortenings, cooking and dietary fats by Ag. TLC/GC. *Ernährungswiss* 34:314–17.

Monardes, N. 1574. *Primera y segunda y tercera partes de la historia medicinal de las cosas que se traen de nuestras Indias Occidentales*. Ed. E. Denot and N. Satanowsky, 1990. Mexico City: Instituto Mexicano de Seguro Social.

Moneret-Vautrin, D. A., G. Kanny, and L. Parisot. 2001. Accidents graves par allergie alimentaire en France: fréquence, caractéristiques cliniques, et idéologiques. Première enquête du Réseau d'allergovigilance, avril–mai 2001. *Revis Français de Allergologie et Immunologie Clinique* 451:696–700.

Mori, T. A., V. Burke, I. B. Puddey, G. F. Watts, D. N. O'Neal, J. D. Best, and L. J. Beilin. 2000. Purified eicosapentaenoic and docosahexaenoic acids have differential effects on serum lipids and lipoproteins, LDL particle size, glucose, and insulin in mildly hyperlipidemic men. *American Journal of Clinical Nutrition* 71:1085–94.

Muggli, R., and P. Clough. 1994. The fats of life. *Roche Magazine* 49:11 pp.

Muir, A. D., and N. D. Westcott. 2000. Quantitation of the lignan secoisolariciresinol diglucoside in baked goods containing flaxseed or flaxmeal. *Journal of Agricultural and Food Chemistry* 48:4048–52.

Munz, P. A., and D. D. Keck. 1959. *A California flora*. Berkeley: University of California Press.

Murthy, H. S. 2002. Indian major carps. In Webster and Lim, 2002:262–72.

Myers, R. A., and B. Worm. 2003. Rapid worldwide depletion of predatory fish communities. *Nature* 423:280–83.

Nabhan, G. P. 1989. *Enduring seeds: native American agriculture and wild plant conservation*. San Francisco: North Point Press.

Nakajima, H. 1996. Siglo XXI: salud para todos. *La Nación* (Buenos Aires, Argentina), 7 October 1996:4.

Nakano, T., M. Sato, and M. Takaeuchi. 1992. Glutathione peroxidase of fish. *Journal of Food Science* 57:1116–19.

Nash, D. M., R. M. G. Hamilton, and H. W. Hulan. 1995. The effect of dietary herring meal on the omega-3 fatty acid content of plasma and egg yolk lipids of laying hens. *Canadian Journal of Animal Science* 75:247–53.

Nash, D. M., R. M. G. Hamilton, K. A. Sanford, and H. W. Hulan. 1996. The effect of dietary menhaden meal and storage on the omega-3 fatty acids and sensory attributes of egg yolk in laying hens. *Canadian Journal of Animal Sciences* 76:377–83.

National Research Council. 1975. *Underexploited tropical plants with promising economic value*. Washington, D.C.: National Academy Press.

———. 1989. *Lost crops of the Incas: little-known plants of the Andes with promise for worldwide cultivation*. Washington, D.C.: National Academy Press.

Naudet, M. 1996. Main chemical constituents of fats: a comprehensive treatise. In Karleskind and Wolff, 1996:67–116.

Neely, E. 1999. Dietary modification of egg yolk lipids. Thesis, School of Agriculture and Food Science, Queen's University of Belfast, Northern Ireland.

Neergaard, L. 2002. Scientific advisers urged government to tell pregnant women to limit how much tuna they eat. Associated Press. 27 July. http://sfgate.com

Nelson, G. J. 1992. Dietary fatty acids and lipid metabolism. In Chow, 1992b:437–71.

Nestle, M. 1995a. Mediterranean diets: historical and research overview. In Nestle, 1995b:1313s–23s.

———, ed. 1995b. Mediterranean diets: science and policy implications. *American Journal of Clinical Nutrition* 61(suppl.).

———. 1995c. Preface. In Nestle, 1995b:ixs–xs.

Nettleton, J. A. 1995. *Omega-3 fatty acids and health*. New York: Chapman and Hall.

Ng, T. K. W., K. Hassan, J. B. Lim, M. S. Lye, and R. Ishak. 1991. Nonhypercholesterolemic effects of a palm-oil diet in Malaysian volunteers. *American Journal of Clinical Nutrition* 53(suppl.):1015s–20s.

Niblo, S. R. 1995. *War, diplomacy, and development: the United States and Mexico*. Wilmington, Del.: Scholarly Resources.

Nishi, K., M. Uno, K. Fukuzawa, H. Horiguchi, K. Shinno, and S. Nagahiro. 2002. Clinicopathological significance of lipid peroxidation in carotid plaques. *Atherosclerosis* 160:289–96.

Nitsan, Z., S. Mokady, and A. Sukenik. 1999. Enrichment of poultry products with omega-3 fatty acids by dietary supplementation with the alga Nannochloropsis and Mantur oil. *Journal of Agricultural and Food Chemistry* 47:5127–32.

Novak, C., and S. Scheideler. 1998. *The effect of calcium and/or vitamin D, supplementation of flax-based diets on production parameters and egg composition*. University of Nebraska Cooperative Extension MP 70, Lincoln.

Odea, K., K. Traianedes, P. Ireland, M. Niall, J. Sadler, J. Hopper, and M. De Luise.

1989. The effects of diet differing in fat, carbohydrate, and fiber on carbohydrate and lipid metabolism in type II diabetes. *Journal of the American Dietetic Association* 89(8):1076–86.

Oh, S. Y., J. Ryue, C. H. Hsieh, and D. E. Bell. 1991. Eggs enriched in omega-3 fatty acids and alterations in lipid concentrations in plasma and lipoproteins and in blood pressure. *American Journal of Clinical Nutrition* 54:689–95.

Okuyama, H. 2001. High n-6 to n-3 ratio of dietary fatty acids rather than serum cholesterol as a major risk factor for coronary heart disease. *European Journal of Lipid Science and Technology* 103:418–22.

Okuyama, H., T. Kobayashi, and S. Watanabe. 1997. Dietary fatty acids: the n-6/n-3 balance and chronic elderly diseases. Excess linoleic acid and relative n-3 deficiency syndrome seen in Japan. *Progress in Lipid Research* 35(4):409–57.

Olivier, J. F. 1996. La vida natural: materias grasas-lípidos. *Aceites y Grasas* 6(22):45–55.

Oomah, B. D., and E. O. Kenaschuk. 1995. Cultivars and agronomic aspects. In Cunnane and Thompson, 1995:43–45.

Organization for Economic Cooperation and Development. 1998. *Towards sustainable development: environmental indicators*. Paris: OECD.

Ortiz de Montellano, B. R. 1978. Aztec cannibalism: an ecological necessity? *Science* 200(4342):611–17.

Palagia, O. 1984. A niche for Kallimachos' lamp? *American Journal of Archaeology* 88:515–21.

Palma, F., M. Donde, and W. R. Lloyd. 1947. Fixed oils of Mexico: I. Oil of chia — *Salvia hispanica*. *Journal of the American Oil Chemists' Society* 24:27–28.

Parmalat. 1999. *Leche plus omega-3*. Parmalat Argentina, Buenos Aires.

Parodi, L. R. 1935. Relaciones de la agricultura prehispánica con la agricultura Argentina actual. *Anales de la Academia Nacional de Agronomía y Veterinaria de Buenos Aires* (Buenos Aires, Argentina) 1:115–67.

Parsons, J. R. 1993. El papel de la agricultura chinampera en el abastecimiento de alimentos de la Tenochtitlán Azteca. In Rojas Rabiela, 1993b:271–300.

Pascual, C., M. M. Esteban, and J. F. Crespo. 1992. Fish allergy: evaluation of the importance of cross-reactivity. *Journal of Pediatrics* 121:S29–34.

Pauletto, P., M. Puato, M. G. Caroli, E. Casiglia, A. E. Munhambo, G. Cazzolato, G. Bittolo Bon, M. T. Angelli, and A. C. Pessina. 1996. Blood pressure and atherogenic lipoprotein profiles of fish-diet and vegetarian villagers in Tanzania: the Lugalawa study. *Lancet* 348:784–88.

Pedersen, A., M. W. Baumstark, P. Markmann, H. Gylling, and B. Sandstrom. 2000. An olive oil—rich diet results in higher concentrations of LDL cholesterol and a higher number of LDL subfraction particles than rapeseed oil and sunflower oil diets. *Journal of Lipid Research* 41:1901–11.

Perrin, M. 2002. Functional foods and nutraceuticals: a recipe for better health. Agriculture and Agro-Food Canada. 8 January. http://www.agr.ca/food/nff/ trnscrpt.html

Perry, M. 1990. *Climate change and world agriculture*. United Nations Environmental Program and the International Institute for Applied Systems Analysis. London: Earthscan Publications Limited.

Pignatelli, P., F. M. Pulcinelli, A. Celestini, L. Lenti, A. Ghiselli, P. P. Gazzaniga, and F. Violi. 2000. The flavonoids quercetin and catechin synergistically inhibit platelet function by antagonizing the intracellular production of hydrogen peroxide. *American Journal of Clinical Nutrition* 72:1150–55.

Planchon, G., and E. Collin. 1895. *Les drogues simples d'origine végétale*. Paris: Octave Doin.

Popper, S. V. 1984. *A reconstruction of Nahua plant classification*. Second Annual Ethnobiology Conference, University of Washington, Seattle, 15–17.

Porsgaard, T., and C. E. Høy. 2000. Lymphatic transport in rats of several dietary fats differing in fatty acid profile and triacyglycerol structure. *Journal of Nutrition* 130:1619–24.

Poulsen, J. B. 1999. *Danish consumers' attitudes towards functional foods*. Aarhus, Denmark: Center of Market Surveillance, Aarhus School of Business, MAPP.

Prescott-Barrows, D. 1971. Desert plant foods of the Coahuila. In *The California Indians*, ed. R. F. Heizer and M. A. Whipple, 306–14. Berkeley: University of California Press.

Ramamoorthy, T. P., R. Bye, A. Lot, and J. Fa, eds. 1993. *Biological diversity of Mexico: origins and distribution*. New York: Oxford University Press.

Ramamoorthy, T. P., and M. Elliot. 1993. Mexican Lamiaceae: diversity, distribution, endemism, and origin. In Ramamoorthy et al., 1993:513–42.

Ratanayake, W. M. N., R. G. Ackman, and H. W. Hulan. 1989. Effect of redfish meal enriched diets on the taste and n-3 PUFAs of 42-day-old broiler chickens. *Journal of the Science of Food and Agriculture* 49:59–74.

Rea, A. de la. 1643. *Crónica de la orden de N. Seráfico P. S. Francisco, provincia de S. Pedro y S. Pablo de Mechoacán en la Nueva España*, ed. Patricia Escandon, 1996. Guadalajara, Mexico: Editorial Gráfica Nueva and Fideicomiso Teixidor.

Reccho, N. A., ed. 1651. *Rerum medicarum Novae Hispaniae thesaurus seu Plantarum animalium mineralium mexicanorum historia*. Rome: Typographeio Vitalis Mascardi.

Redfield, M. P. 1929. Notes on the cookery of Tepoztlan, Morelos. *Journal of American Folklore* 42(164):167–96.

Renaud, S., M. de Lorgeril, J. Delaye, J. Guidollet, F. Jacquard, N. Mamelle, J. L. Martin, I. Monjaud, P. Salen, and P. Toubel. 1995. Cretan Mediterranean diet for prevention of coronary heart disease. In Nestle, 1995b:1360s–96s.

Rickard, S. E., and L. U. Thompson. 1988. Chronic exposure to secoisolariciresinol diglycosede alters lignin disposition in rats. *Journal of Nutrition* 128(3):615–23.

Ridges, L., R. Sunderland, K. Moerman, B. Meyer, L. Astheimer, and P. Howe. 2001. Cholesterol lowering benefits of soy and linseed enriched foods. *Asian Pacific Journal of Nutrition* 10(3):204–11.

Robbelen, G., R. K. Downey, and A. Ashri. 1989. *Oil crops of the world*. New York: McGraw-Hill.

Robinson, E. H., and M. H. Li. 2002. Channel catfish, *Ictalurus punctatus*. In Webster and Lim, 2002:293–318.

Rodríguez Vallejo, J. 1992. *Historia de la agricultura y de la fitopatología, con referencia especial a México*. Mexico City: Colegio de Post-graduados en Ciencias Agrícolas.

Rojas Rabiela, T. 1991. Raíces históricas de las técnicas y conocimientos agrícolas novohispanos. In Universidad Autónoma Chapingo, 1992:113–20.

———. 1993a. Evolución histórica del repertorio de plantas cultivadas en las chinampas de la cuenca de México. In Rojas Rabiela, 1993b:203–51.

———, ed. 1993b. *La agricultura chinampera: compilación histórica*. Chapingo, Mexico: Universidad Autónoma Chapingo.

Rose, D. P., and J. M. Connolly. 2000. Regulation of tumor angiogenesis by dietary fatty acids and eicosanoids. *Nutrition and Cancer* 37(2):119–27.

Rulfo, J. M. 1937. La chía. *Agricultura* 1:28–37.

Rzedowski, J. 1978. *Vegetación de México*. Mexico City: Editorial Limusa.

Sacks, F. M. 1998. Scientific basis of the healthy Mediterranean diet. *Australian Journal of Nutrition and Dietetics* 55(4 suppl.):s4–s7.

Sahagún, B. de 1579. *Historia general de las cosas de Nueva España* (Codex Florentino). Ed. A. M. Garibay, 1989. Mexico City: Editorial Porrua.

Sanders, W. T. 1976. The agricultural history of the Basin of Mexico. In *The Valley of Mexico*, ed. E. R. Wolf, 101–59. Albuquerque: University of New Mexico Press.

Saouma, E. 1992. Preámbulo. In *Cultivos marginados: otra perspectiva de 1492*, ed. J. E. Hernández Bermejo and J. León, v–vi. Organización para la Agricultura y la Alimentación, Producción y Protección Vegetal No. 26.

Sargent, J., G. Bell, L. McEvoy, D. Tocher, and A. Estevez. 1999. Recent developments in the essential fatty acids nutrition of fish. *Aquaculture* 77:191–99.

Sauer, J. D. 1950. The grain amaranths: a survey of their history and classification. *Annals of the Missouri Botanical Garden* 37(4):113–25.

Saunders, C. F. 1920. *Useful wild plants of the United States and Canada*. New York: Robert M. McBride and Company.

Schaefer, E. J., A. H. Lichtenstein, S. Lamon-Fava, J. H. Contois, Z. Li, B. R. Goldin, H. Rasmussen, J. R. McNamara, and J. M. Ordovas. 1996. Effects of national cholesterol education program step 2 diets relatively high or relatively low in fish-derived fatty acids on plasma lipoproteins in middle-aged and elderly subjects. *American Journal of Clinical Nutrition* 63:234–41.

Schaefer, E. J., A. H. Lichtenstein, S. Lamon-Fava, J. R. McNamara, and J. M. Ordovas. 1995. Lipoproteins, nutrition, aging, and atherosclerosis. *American Journal of Clinical Nutrition* 61(suppl.):726s–40s.

Scheideler, S. E., G. Froning, and S. Cuppett. 1997. Studies of consumer acceptance of high omega-3 fatty acid—enriched eggs. *Journal of Applied Poultry Research* 6:137–46.

Schery, R. W. 1972. *Plants for man.* Englewood Cliffs, N.J.: Prentice-Hall.

Schilling, E. 1993. Los jardines flotantes de Xochimilco. In Rojas Rabiela, 1993b:77–109.

Schmidt, D. B. 2000. Consumer response to functional foods. *AgBioForum* 3:266–71.

Schonfeld, R. 2002. National survey reports high consumer awareness of omega-3. Omega Protein, Inc. 2 April. http://www.omega-pure.com

Scott, T. W., L. J. Cook, and S. C. Mills. 1971. Protection of dietary polyunsaturated fatty acids against microbial hydrogenation in ruminants. *Journal of the American Oil Chemists' Society* 48:358–64.

Sebedio, J. L. 1995. Marine oils. In Karleskind and Wolff, 1996:266–99.

Selhub, J., P. Jaques, A. Bostom, R. D'Agostino, P. Wilson, A. Belanger, D. Oleary, P. Wolf, D. Rush, E. Schefer, and I. Rosenberg. 1996. Relationship between plasma homocysteine, vitamin status and extracranial carotid-artery stenosis in the Framingham study population. *Journal of Nutrition* 126:1258s–65s.

Sheehy, P. J. A., and P. A. Morrissey. 1998. Functional foods: prospects and perspectives. In *Nutritional aspects of food processing and ingredients*, ed. C. J. K. Henry and N. J. Heppell, 45–65. Gaithersburg, Md.: Aspen Publishers.

Shreve, F., and I. Wiggins. 1986. *Vegetation and flora of the Sonoran desert.* Stanford, Calif.: Stanford University Press.

Shukla, V. K. S., P. K. J. P. D. Wanasundra, and F. Shahidi. 1996. Natural antioxidants from oilseeds. In *Natural antioxidants*, ed. F. Shahidi, 97–132. Champaign, Ill.: American Oil Chemists' Society Press.

Sibbald, I. R. 1975. The effect of level of feed intake on metabolizable energy values measured with adult roosters. *Poultry Science* 54:1990–97.

Siguel, E. 1996. Issues and problems in the design of foods rich in essential fatty acids. *Lipid Technology Newsletter* 8(4):81–86.

Sim, J. S., and Z. Jiang. 1994. Consumption of omega-3 PUFAs enriched eggs and changes of plasma lipids in human subjects. In *Egg uses and processing technologies: new developments*, ed. J. S. Sim and S. Nakai, 414–20. Wallingford, Oxfordshire, U.K.: CAB International.

Sim, J. S., S. Nakai, and W. Guenter, eds. 2000. *Egg nutrition and technology*. Wallingford, Oxfordshire, U.K.: CAB International.

Simon, J. A., J. Fong, J. T. Bernert, and W. S. Browner. 1995. Serum fatty acids and the risk of stroke. *Stroke* 26:778–82.

Simopoulos, A. P. 1988. Executive summary. In Galli and Simopoulos, 1988:391–402.

———. 1998a. Overview of evolutionary aspects of omega-3 fatty acids in the diet. In Simopoulos, 1998b:1–11.

———, ed. 1998b. *The return of omega-3 fatty acids into the food supply*. Basel, Switzerland: Karger AG.

———. 1999a. Essential fatty acids in health and chronic disease. *American Journal of Clinical Nutrition* 70(3):560s–69s.

———. 1999b. Genetic variation and nutrition. In *Evolutionary aspects of nutrition and health: diet, exercise, genetics and chronic disease*, ed. A. P. Simopoulos. *World Review of Nutrition and Dietetics* 84:118–40.

———. 2001. The Mediterranean diets: what is so special about the diet of Greece? The scientific evidence. *Journal of Nutrition* 131:3065s–73s.

———. 2002. Omega-3 fatty acids in wild plants, nuts and seeds. *Asia Pacific Journal of Clinical Nutrition* 11(6):s163–s173.

———. 2003. Common statement. In *First international congress on the Columbus concept*, ed. F. De Meester. Bastogne, Belgium: Belovo SA.

Simopoulos, A. P., A. Leaf, and N. Salem. 2000. Workshop on the essentiality of and recommended dietary intakes for omega-6 and omega-3 fatty acids. *Food Review International* 16(1):113–17.

Simopoulos, A. P., and N. Salem Jr. 1992. Egg yolk as a source of long-chain polyunsaturated fatty acids in infant feeding. *American Journal of Clinical Nutrition* 55:411–14.

Simopoulos, A. P., and F. Visioli. 2000. Mediterranean diets. *World Review of Nutrition and Dietetics* 87:1–184.

Sinclair, A. J., K. S. Oon, L. Lim, D. Li, and N. J. Mann. 1998. The omega-3 fatty acid content of canned, smoked and fresh fish in Australia. *Australian Journal of Nutritional Diet* 55(3):116–20.

Sloan, A. E. 1998. Food industry forecast: consumer trends to 2020 and beyond. *Food Technology* 52(1):37–44.

———. 1999. The new market: food for the not-so-healthy. *Food Technology* 53(2):54–60.

Smith, D., G. Song, and T. Sheldon. 1993. Cholesterol lowering and mortality: the importance of considering initial level of risk. *British Medical Journal* 306:1367–73.

Smith, G., M. Shipley, M. Marmot, and G. Rose. 1992. Plasma cholesterol concentration and mortality: The Whitehall study. *Journal of the American Medical Association* 267:70–76.

Solbrig, O. T., and D. J. Solbrig. 1990. No small potatoes: the importance of crops in history. Harvard University, Boston, Mass.

Solís, A. de. 1770. *Historia de la conquista de México, población y progresos de la América septentrional, conocida por el nombre de Nueva España.* Barcelona: Francisco Oliver y Marti.

Song, J. H., K. Fujimoto, and T. Miyazawa. 2000. Polyunsaturated (n-3) fatty acids susceptible to peroxidation are increased in plasma and tissue lipids of rats fed docosahexaenoic acid—containing oils. *Journal of Nutrition* 130:3028–33.

Song, J. H., and T. Miyazawa. 2001. Enhanced level of n-3 fatty acid in membrane phospholipids induces lipid peroxidation in rats fed dietary docosahexaenoic acid oil. *Atherosclerosis* 155:9–18.

Soustelle, J. 1955. *La vie quotidienne des aztèques à la veille de la conquête espagnole.* Paris: Hachette.

Steinberg, D., and A. M. Gotto. 1999. Preventing coronary artery disease by lowering cholesterol levels. *Journal of the American Medical Association* 282(21):2043–50.

Stitt, P. A. 1988. Flax as a source of alpha-linolenic acid. In Galli and Simopoulos, 1988:389–90.

Straarup, E. M., and C. E. Høy. 2000. Structured lipids improve fat absorption in normal and malabsorbing rats. *Journal of Nutrition* 130:2802–8.

Sultana, C. 1996. Oleaginous flax. In Karleskind and Wolff, 1996:157–60.

Svensson, B. G., A. Nilsson, M. Hansson, C. Rappe, B. Akesson, and S. Skerfving. 1991. Exposure to dioxins and dibenzofurans through the consumption of fish. *New England Journal of Medicine* 32(1):8–12.

Taga, M. S., E. E. Miller, and D. E. Pratt, 1984. Chia seeds as a source of natural lipid antioxidants. *Journal of the American Oil Chemists' Society* 61:928–31.

Talha, M., and F. Osman. 1975. Effect of soil water stress on water economy and oil composition in sunflower. *Journal of Agriculture Science* 84:49–56.

Taraszewaski, A., and G. L. Jensen. 1994. N-6 fatty acids. In Forse, 1994:165–78.

Taylor-Chinn, M. 2000. Homocysteine and arteriosclerotic heart disease. *Clinician Reviews* 10(10):45–57.

Temme, E., R. Mensink, and G. Hornstra. 1994. Effects of lauric and palmitic acid on serum lipids. *Voeding* 55:32.

Tengerdy, R. P., and J. C. Brown. 1977. Effect of vitamin E and A on humoral immunity and phagocytosis in *E. coli* infected chicken. *Poultry Science* 56:957–63.

Thies, F., G. Nebe-von Caron, J. R. Powel, P. Yagoob, E. A. Newsholme, and P. Calder. 2001. Dietary supplementation with eiosapentaenoic acid, but not with other long-chain n-3 or n-6 polyunsaturated fatty acids, decreases natural killer cell activity in healthy subjects aged >55 y. *American Journal of Clinical Nutrition* 73:539–48.

Thomsen, M. K., C. Jacobsen, and L. Skibsted. 2000. Initiation mechanisms of oxidation in fish oil enriched mayonnaise. *European Food Research and Technology* 211:381–86.

Ting, I. P., J. H. Brown, H. H. Naqvi, J. Kumamoto, and M. Matsumura. 1990. Chia: a potential oil crop for arid zones. In *New industrial crops and products: proceedings of the first international conference on new industrial crops and products*, ed. H. H. Naqvi, A. Estilai, and I. P. Ting, 197–202. Riverside, Calif.: Association for the Advancement of Industrial Crops.

Tornaritis, M., E. Peraki, M. Georgulli, A. Kafatos, G. Charalambbakis, P. Divanack, M. Kentouri, S. Yiannopoulos, H. Frenaritou, and R. Argyrides. 1994. Fatty acid composition and total fat content of eight species of Mediterranean fish. *International Journal of Food Sciences and Nutrition* 45:135–39.

Torquemada, J. de. 1615. *Veinte i un libros rituales i monarquía indiana con el origen y guerras de los indios ocidentales de sus poblaciones descubrimiento, conquista, conversion y otras cosas maravillosas de la mesma tierra distrybuidos en tres tomos*. Pt. 2. Office and *acosta* by Nicolas Rodríguez Franco, 1723. Madrid.

Torres, B. 1985. Las plantas útiles en el México antiguo según las fuentes del siglo XVI. In *Historia de la agricultura epoca prehispánica siglo XVI*, ed. T. Rojas Rabiela and W. T. Sanders, 53–58. Mexico City: Instituto Nacional de Antropología e Historia.

Toug, J. C., J. Chen, and L. U. Thompson. 1998. Flaxseed and its lignan precursor secoisolariciresinol diglycoside affect pregnancy outcome and reproductive development in rats. *Journal of Nutrition* 128(11):1861–68.

Treviño, J., M. L. Rodríguez, L. T. Ortiz, A. Rebole, and C. Alzueta. 2000. Protein quality of linseed for growing broiler chicks. *Animal Food Science and Technology* 84:155–66.

Truelsen, S. 1999. Functional foods are big in Ag's future. *Voice of Agriculture* 78:33. American Farm Bureau Federation. 12 December 2001. http://www.fb.com/news/fbn/99/09_13/html/functional.html

Turini, M. E., W. S. Powell, S. R. Behr, and B. J. Holub. 1994. Effects of a fish-oil and vegetable-oil formula on an aggregation and ethanolamine-containing lysophospholipid generation in activated human platelets and on leukotriene production in stimulated neutrophils. *American Journal of Clinical Nutrition* 60:717–24.

Tylor, E. 1993. Fragmento sobre las chinampas. In Rojas Rabiela, 1993b:41–42.

Ucciani, E. 1995. *Nouveau dictionnaire des huiles végétales: compositions en acides gras*. Paris: Lavoisier.

United Nations. 1990. *Perspectivas socioeconómicas generales de la economía mundial hasta el año 2000*. New York: Naciones Unidas.

References   183

United States Department of Agriculture. 1943. *Economic plants of interest to the Americas: citicica and chia oils*. Office of Foreign Agricultural Relations.

———. 1988. *Alternative opportunities for U.S. farmers*. Washington, D.C.: Cooperative State Research Service.

———. 1996a. *Agricultural statistics 1995–96*. Washington, D.C.: United States Government Printing Office.

———. 1996b. *Long-term agricultural projections to 2005*. World Agricultural Outlook Board, Office of the Chief Economist, Staff Report No. WAOB-96-1, Washington, D.C.

———. 1997. Data tables: intakes of 19 individual fatty acids; results from *1994–96 continuing survey of food intakes by individuals*. Agricultural Research Service, Food Surveys Research Group. 2 November 2000. http://www.bar.usda.gov/foodsurvey/home.htm

———. 1998. *Agricultural statistics 1998*. Washington, D.C.: United States Government Printing Office.

———. 1999. USDA nutrient database for standard reference, release 13. Agricultural Research Service, Nutrient Data Laboratory Home Page. 26 March 2001. http://www.nal.usda.gov/fnic/foodcomp

———. 2000. *Report of the dietary guidelines advisory committee on the dietary guidelines for Americans, 2000*. Dietary Guidelines Advisory Committee, Agricultural Research Service, Washington, D.C.

———. 2001. USDA nutrient database for standard reference, release 14. Agricultural Research Service, Nutrient Data Laboratory Home Page. 11 March. http://www.nal.usda.gov/fnic/foodcomp

———. 2002. USDA nutrient database for standard reference, release 15. Agricultural Research Service, Nutrient Data Laboratory Home Page. http://www.nal.usda.gov/fnic/foodcomp

———. 2003. USDA nutrient database for standard reference, release 16. Agricultural Research Service, Nutrient Data Laboratory Home Page. 12 March. http://www.nal.usda.gov/fnic/foodcomp/

United States Department of Agriculture and United States Department of Health and Human Services. 1995. *Nutrition and your health: dietary guidelines for Americans*. Home and Garden Bulletin No. 232, 4th ed. Washington, D.C.

United States Department of Health and Human Services. 1999. *Chronic diseases and their risk factors: the nation's leading causes of death*. Atlanta: Centers for Disease Control and Prevention.

Universidad Autónoma Chapingo, ed. 1992. *Agricultura y agronomía en México*. Chapingo, Mexico.

Valenzuela, A., and R. Uauy. 1999. Consumption pattern of dietary fats in Chile: n-6 and n-3 fatty acids. *International Journal of Food Sciences and Nutrition* 50:127–33.

Vander Jagt, D. J., C. D. Arndt, S. N. Okolo, Y. S. Huang, L. T. Chuang, and R. H. Glew. 2000. Fatty acid composition of the milk lipid of Fulani women and the serum phospholipids of their exclusively breast-fed infants. *Early Human Development* 60:73–87.

Van Elswyk, M. E., P. L. Dawson, and A. R. Sams. 1995. Dietary menhaden oil influences sensory characteristics and head space volatiles of shell eggs. *Journal of Food Science* 60:85–89.

Van Elswyk, M. E., B. M. Hargis, J. D. Williams, and P. S. Hargis. 1994. Dietary menhaden oil contributes to hepatic lipidosis in laying hens. *Poultry Science* 73:653–62.

Van Elswyk, M. E., S. D. Hatch, G. G. Stella, P. K. Mayo, and K. S. Kubena. 1998. Poultry-based alternatives for enhancing the omega-3 fatty acid content of American diets. In Simopoulos, 1998b:103–15.

———. 2000. Eggs as functional foods alternative to fish and supplements for the consumption of DHA. In Sim, Nakai, and Guenter, 2000:121–33.

Van Elswyk, M. E., A. R. Sams, and P. S. Hargis. 1992. Composition, functionality, and sensory evaluation of eggs from hens fed dietary menhaden oil. *Journal of Food Science* 57:342–49.

Variyam, J. N. 1999. Role of demographics, knowledge, and attitudes. In *America's eating habits: changes and consequences*, ed. E. Frazao, 281–94. United States Department of Agriculture, Agriculture Information Bulletin No. 750.

Vavilov, N. I. 1931. Mexico and Central America as the principal entré of the origin of cultivated plants of the New World. *Bulletin of Applied Botany, Genetic and Plant Breeding* 26(3):135–99.

Vergara Santana, M. I., S. Lemus Juárez, and R. Bayardo Parra. 2001. Caracterización botánica-agronómica de *Hyptis suaveolens* Chiantzotzolli: la chía que formó parte del complejo huautli-chian en la época prehispánica de México. In *Abstracts of the XV congreso mexicano de botánica — etnobotánica*. Queretaro, Mexico: Sociedad Botánica de México.

Verschuren, M., D. Jacobs, B. Bloemberg, H. Kromhout, A. Menotti, C. Aravanis, H. Blackburn, N. Buzina, A. Dontas, F. Fidanza, M. Karvonen, F. Nedeljkovic, A. Nissinen, and H. Toshima. 1995. Serum total cholesterol and long-term coronary heart disease mortality in different cultures. *Journal of the American Medical Association* 274(2):131–36.

Vetter, J. 2000. Plant cyanogenetic glycosides. *Toxicon* 38:11–36.

Vietmeyer, N. D. 1978. Neglected riches of nature. In *The Smithsonian book of invention*. Washington, D.C.: Smithsonian Exposition Books.

von Sharky, C., P. Angerer, W. Kothny, K. Theisen, and H. Mudra. 1999. The effect of dietary omega-3 fatty acids on coronary atherosclerosis. *Annals of Internal Medicine* 130:554–62.

von Wullerstorff, B. 1990. Outlook for oleochemicals in Europe. In Bont, 1990:2–9.
Wadley, G., and A. Martin. 1993. The origins of agriculture: a biological perspective and a new hypothesis. *Australian Biologist* 6:96–105.
Wander, R. C., J. A. Hall, J. L. Gradin, S. H. Du, and D. E. Jewell. 1997. The ratio of dietary (n-6) to (n-3) fatty acids influences immune system function, eicosanoid metabolism, lipid peroxidation and vitamin E status in aged dogs. *Journal of Nutrition* 127:1198–205.
Watanabe, F., M. Goto, K. Abe, and Y. Nakano. 1996. Glutathione peroxidase activity during storage of fish muscle. *Journal of Food Science* 61:734–35.
Watson, G. 1938. Nahuatl word in American English. *American Speech* 13(2):108–21.
Weber, C. W., H. S. Gentry, E. A. Kohlhepp, and P. R. McCrohan. 1991. The nutritional and chemical evaluation of chia seeds. *Ecology of Food and Nutrition* 26:119–25.
Webster, C. D., and C. Lim, eds. 2002. *Nutrient requirements and feeding of finfish for aquaculture.* Wallingford, Oxfordshire, U.K.: CAB International.
Welch, V. A., and J. T. Borlakoglu. 1992. Absorption and transport of dietary lipid: effect of some lipid-related health problems. In Chow, 1992b:559–630.
White, P. J. 1992. Fatty acids in oilseeds (vegetable oil). In Chow, 1992b:237–62.
Whitmore, T. M., and B. L. Turner II. 1992. Landscapes of cultivation in Mesoamerica on the eve of the conquest. *Annals of the Association of American Geographers* 82(3):402–25.
Wilkes, J. G., E. D. Conte, Y. Kim, M. Holcomb, J. B. Sutherland, and D. W. Miller. 2000. Sample preparation for the analysis of flavors and off-flavors in foods. *Journal of Chromatography A* 880:3–33.
Willet, W. C., F. Sacks, A. Trichopoulou, G. Drescher, A. Ferro-Luzzi, E. Helsing, and D. Trichopoulous. 1995. Mediterranean diet pyramid: a cultural model for healthy eating. In Nestle, 1995b:1402s–6s.
Williams, P. T. 1996. HDL-cholesterol level increased by exercise. *New England Journal of Medicine* 334:1298–303.
Williard, D. E., S. D. Harmon, T. I. Kaduce, M. Preuss, S. A. Moore, M. E. C. Robbins, and A. A. Spector. 2001. DHA synthesis from n-3 polyunsaturated fatty acids in differentiated rat brain astrocytes. *Journal of Lipid Research* 42:1368–376.
Wilson, E. O. 1988. The current state of biological diversity. In *Bio-diversity*, ed. E. O. Wilson and F. M. Peter, 3–18. Washington, D.C.: National Academy Press.
Wilson, R. F., J. W. Burton, and C. A. Brim. 1981. Progress in the selection for altered fatty acid composition in soybeans. *Crop Science* 21:788–91.
Wimmer, A. 2001. Dictionnaire de la langue nahuatl classique. 16 September. http://www.ifrance.com/nahuatl
Wood, P. J., J. W. Anderson, J. R. Braaten, N. A. Cave, F. W. Scott, and C. Vachon.

1989. Physiological effects of beta D glucan rich fractions from oats. *Cereals Food World* 34(10):878–82.

World Health Organization. 1995. The world health report 1995: bridging the gaps. *World Health Forum* 16:377–85.

———. 2003. *Diet, nutrition and the prevention of chronic diseases.* Report of a joint WHO/Food and Agriculture Organization Expert Consultation, WHO Technical Report Series 916, World Health Organization, Geneva, Switzerland.

Worsley, A., and V. Scott. 2000. Consumers' concerns about food and health in Australia and New Zealand. *Asia Pacific Journal of Clinical Nutrition* 9(1):24–32.

Wright, C. 2000. Mercadeo de huevos omega-3 en Brasil. *Industria Avicola*, 7–10.

Wright, T. C., S. Moscardini, P. H. Luimes, P. Susmel, and B. W. McBride. 1998. Effects of rumen-undegradable protein and feed intake on milk protein production and nitrogen balance in dairy cows. *Journal of Dairy Science* 81:784–87.

Wu, D., and S. N. Meydani. 1998. N-3 polyunsaturated fatty acids and immune function. *Proceedings of the Nutrition Society* 57:503–9.

Yli-Jama, P., T. S. Haugen, H. M. Rebnord, J. Ringstad, and J. I. Pedersen. 2001. Selective mobilization of fatty acids from human adipose tissue. *European Journal of Internal Medicine* 12:107–15.

Yonekubo, A., Y. Katoku, T. Kanno, M. Yamada, T. Kuwata, A. Sawa, and A. Kobayashi. 1998. Effects of cholesterol and nucleotide in infant formula on lipid composition of plasma and red blood cell membrane in early infancy. In Huang and Sinclair, 1998:156–67.

Young, J. 1997. Functional foods market still to grow. *Food Ingredients and Analysis International* 19:43–57.

Zlotkin, S. H. 1996. A review of the Canadian nutrition recommendations update: dietary fat and children. *Journal of Nutrition* 126:1022s–27s.

Zuaza, F. de. 1689. *Descripción geográfico-moral de la Diócesis de Goathemala.* Vol. 20. Guatemala City: Sociedad de Geográfica e Historia de Guatemala.

INDEX

AA. *See* arachidonic acid
Abrams, Barbara, 16
Acatic, 80, 82, 99, 101, 102, 104, 108
agriculture: agronomic aspects of, 101–4;
  demonstration projects, 83–85; and food
  access, 7–8; Mesoamerican, 44, 47–53, 80;
  in Peru, 5–6; production, 1–2, 99–107;
  overproduction, 3–4; specialization in,
  4–5
agrochemicals, 3, 8
agua de chía, 74, 79
Alauiztla, 65
alegría, 66
algae: marine, 109, 110(table), 111, 126, 132
allergins: food, 112, 122
alpha-linolenic acid, 22, 29–30, 31, 32–33,
  40–41, 109, 112, 114, 125
AMACUP. *See* Asociación Mexicana de
  Arte y Cultural Popular
amaranth, 56, 65–66, 75, 77
Amaranthus, 56, 65–66, 75, 77, 89;
  leucocarpus, 91(table), 97–98

American Association of Cereal Chemists,
  119
amino acids, 114–15
Anderson, Arthur J. O., 57
animal feed: cattle, 137–38; horses, 140;
  poultry, 127–30, 133–37
animal products, 12–13
animals: as food source, 13–14
"Antigüedades de la Nueva España"
  (Hernández), 46, 66
antioxidants, 31, 41, 117–19, 126, 129
aquaculture, 124, 125–26
arachidonic acid (AA), 22
Argentina, 4, 23, 121, 136, 143; chia
  production in, 83–84, 89, 96, 101, 102,
  103, 104, 106(table), 107, 108, 113(table),
  114, 120, 140; egg use in, 127,
  146–47(table); milk production in, 138,
  144, 148(table)
Argentina Celiac Association, 114
Argentine National Institute of Agricultural
  Technology (INTA), 136

Arizona, 78, 85, 97, 108, 139, 140
Asociación Mexicana de Arte y Cultura
    Popular (AMACUP), 73
atolli chiampitzahuac, 66
Australia, 142–43
Azcaputzaleas, 59
Aztecs, 55(fig.), 56; botanical gardens of,
    62–63; chia use by, 10, 43, 58–60, 63–73,
    145, 148–49; cropping system of, 48–50;
    food shortages among, 51–52; historical
    records of, 45–47, 53–54; Huitzilopochtli
    ceremonies and, 76–77; knowledge of,
    57–58

Badiano, Juan, 59
Baja California, 78, 97
Beaumont, Pablo de la Purísma
    Concepción, 72
Belgium, 121, 143, 144, 146–47(table),
    148(table)
Belize, 44
Benavente, Toribio de, 89
beverages, 66, 68, 74, 92, 93, 139
biodiversity, 8–9
Bolivia, 84, 89, 99, 101, 102, 103, 107,
    113(table)
Bourlag, Norman, 1 botanical classification:
    of chia, 89–97; Nahua system of, 87–88
botanical gardens: Nahua, 62–63
Brazil, 4, 138, 143
British Nutrition Foundation, 32, 34, 36, 38,
    138

caffeic acid, 117
California, 70, 78, 89, 97, 120, 139, 140
calories, 20, 26–27
Canada, 26–27, 36, 124, 125, 140, 141, 142,
    143
cancer, 117–18, 125
Carrefour, 140
cassava (*Manihot esculenta* C.), 4
Castro, Fidel, 77
Catamarca, 83, 85

Catholicism, 54, 75, 76–77
Cauca, Valle de, 85, 102, 104, 108
celiac disease, 114
Center for Genetics, Nutrition and
    Health, 13
Centers for Disease Control, 16
Central Valley of Mexico, 44, 45, 49, 51, 104,
    108
cereals, 1–2, 4, 9, 15, 119, 145
Cervantes de Salazar, Francisco, 60, 65,
    71, 93
Charles I, 45
CHD. *See* coronary heart disease
chia, 10, 100; classification of, 89, 98;
    descriptions of, 93–94; post-conquest use
    of, 75, 79–85; pre-Columbian use of,
    64–65, wrinkled, 90. *See also Hyptis
    suaveolens*; *Salvia columbariae*; *S. hispanica*
chía de chapata, 97
chía de Colima (*Hyptis suaveolens*), 94
chía fresca, 66, 78, 139
chía gorda (*Hyptis suaveolens*), 94
chiamatl, 71
chian, (*Salvia hispanica L.*), 89, 90
chianatolli, 66
chian mazamorra, 68
chianpinolli, 66
chianpitzaoal, 89
chiantzotzoatolli, 93
chiantzotzotl (*Hyptis suaveolens*), 90, 92,
    93, 94
Chiapanecas, 74
Chiapas, 72, 73–74
Chia Pets, 139
chía pinta, 108
chía poblana, 108
chickens: diets for, 128–37, 140
Chiepetlán, 80
Chile, 125
China, 32
chinampas, 46, 48–49, 79, 154
chlorogenic acid, 117
Choele-Choel, 104

cholesterol, 26, 38, 118, 123; and coronary heart disease, 24–25, 40; oleic acid and, 27–28

Chontales, 74

Ciudad Real, Antonio de, 79

Clavijero, Francisco Javier, 60, 68, 78, 93–94

climate: and agricultural production, 49–52, 101, 102

Coahuila (people), 97

cod liver oil, 123, 130

Codex Badianus (Barberini), 59–60, 70

Codex Borbonicus, 53

Codex Florentino, 56–58, 59, 71, 77, 89, 97, 108; on chia as food, 66, 68, 69; chia classification in, 90, 92–93

Codex Mendocino, 54

Codex Mendoza, 54, 56, 59, 65

codices, 53–54

Colima, 93, 94

Colombia, 4, 85, 99, 102, 103, 104, 107, 108, 113(table)

Columbus, Christopher, 45

Copan, 47, 74

coronary heart disease (CHD), 23, 117, 121, 127; cholesterol and, 24–25; fatty acids and, 25–27, 28–36, 132; Mediterranean diet and, 38–41

Cortés, Hernán, 45–46, 60

Cortés, Martín, 60

Cortés y Larraz, Pedro, 79

cosmetics, 71

Costa Rica, 44

cows, 137–38

CREA Los Lapachos growers group, 83

Crete, 27, 39, 40

Croatia-Serbia, 24

Crónica de la Nueva España (Cervantes de Salazar), 60, 65, 71

Crónica de la orden de N. Seráfico P. S. Francisco, provincia de S. Pedro y S. Pablo de Mechoacán en la Nueva España (Rea), 71–72

Crónica de Mechoacán (Beaumont), 72

cropping system: Mesoamerican, 48–51, 52–53

crops, 1, 57(table), 65, 99; diversity of, 8–9; Mesoamerican, 54, 56, 146, 148–49; New World, 9–10; post-conquest, 75–78, 80; production of, 2–3, 84–85

Cruz, Martín de la, 59

Cultural Bancomer Foundation, 73

culture: Mesoamerican, 44–47

demonstration projects, 83–84

Denmark, 143

Department of Health and Welfare (Canada), 36

dependence: food, 5, 15

desaturation, 22, 35, 125

DHA. *See* docasahexaenoic acid

diabetes, 15, 119

Díaz del Castillo, Bernal, 75

Dibble, Charles, 57

diclycoside ecoisolariciresinol (SDG), 121

diet, 5, 37(table); chia in, 63, 145, 148–49; and disease, 15, 25–27; and fatty acids, 29–36; and human evolution, 11–14; Hispanic, 16–17; Mediterranean, 38–40; poultry, 129, 133–34, 135, 136–37

diseases, 15, 103; antioxidants and, 117–18; cardiovascular, 22–23; fatty acids and, 17–18. *See also* coronary heart disease

diversity, 8, 9; diet, 16–17; Lamiaceae, 98–99

docosahexaenoic acid (DHA), 22, 28, 29, 123, 125, 126; and alpha-linolenic acid, 32–33; hydrogenation and, 38, 122; sources of, 30–31, 109

domestication: diet and, 13–14; plant, 47, 61

Dos libros (Monardes), 61

drinks, 66, 68

drought, 50, 51

Durán, Diego, 59, 65, 68–69

eggs, 131(table), 140; omega-3 enriched, 127–28, 129–30, 143–44, 146–47(table)

ABOUT THE AUTHORS

Ricardo Ayerza Jr. is an Associate in Arid Lands in the Office of Arid Lands Studies at the University of Arizona. A native of Buenos Aires, he has authored numerous scientific articles and three books on new crops. He has been doing research on chia production and utilization since 1990. He is also working on selection and production of chia lines for different environments.

Wayne Coates is Professor Emeritus in the Office of Arid Lands Studies at the University of Arizona. He is the author of more than 60 articles in technical journals. His work with chia began in 1990, and he developed the system that is now used to harvest and clean the seed. His current research activites are focused on making this healthy seed widely known and used throughout the world.

Library of Congress Cataloging-in-Publication Data
Ayerza, Ricardo, 1951–
Chia : rediscovering a forgotten crop of the Aztecs /
Ricardo Ayerza, Jr. and Wayne Coates.
p. cm.
Includes bibliographical references and index.
ISBN 0-8165-2488-2 (pbk. : alk. paper)
ISBN 0-8165-2438-6 (cloth : alk. paper)
1. Chia. 1. Coates, Wayne, 1947– II. Title.
SB299.C5A94 2005
635'.6—dc22
2004023863